# Curious, Odd, &

T0119254

# Abnormal
# Reactions
# to
# Medications

# Curious, Odd, Rare,
# &
# Abnormal
# Reactions
# to
# Medications

by

Jerome Z. Litt, MD

Published by Barricade Books Inc.
185 Bridge Plaza North
Suite 308-A
Fort Lee, NJ 07024

www.barricadebooks.com

ISBN 13: 978-1-56980-367-7
ISBN 1-56980-367-6

Library of Congress Cataloging-in-Publication Data

Litt, Jerome Z.
  Curious, odd, rare, and abnormal reactions to medications / by Jerome Z. Litt.
    p. cm.
  ISBN 978-1-56980-367-7
1. Drug allergy—Popular works. I. Title.

  RC598.D7L58 2009
  616.97—dc22

2008051048

10 9 8 7 6 5 4 3 2 1

Manufactured in the United States of America

*To Vel,*

*My Muse*

# TABLE OF CONTENTS

# Part B - Skin And Hair Disorders

# Part C - Mouth/Tongue/Teeth/ Gum Disorders

# Part D - Hearing Disorders

# ACKNOWLEDGMENTS

I am grateful to the many people who have helped me in this labor of love, not the least of whom has been my bride for the past thirty-five years who has been a great inspiration for me . . .

Several books have helped me direct my writings:

*Musicophilia*, by the author/neurologist, Dr. Oliver Sacks

*Smell*, by Piet Vroon

*The Dirt on Clean*, by Katherine Ashenburg

*Dreams and Dreaming*, Time-Life Books

*Keeping Clean*, by Daisy Kerr

*Drug Eruption Reference Manual*, Jerome Z. Litt

*Your Skin From A to Z*, Jerome Z. Litt

In addition, Wikipedia, Answers.com, and the entire Internet have been invaluable sources for much of the technical information herein.

Jerome Z. Litt, MD

# INTRODUCTION

## Adverse Drug Reactions

"Any side effect can be due to any drug."

It is an inescapable truth that more and more people—primarily the elderly—are taking increasingly more over-the-counter and prescription medications. New drugs for all types of disorders—high blood pressure, stomach ulcers, diabetes, high cholesterol, and so forth—are appearing in the medical marketplace on an almost daily basis; and there are more than 1,800 new drugs in the pipeline at any one time. Unfortunately, more and more adverse drug reactions have been arising from many of these medications.

In the course of writing a technical treatise for fifteen years, updated yearly, relating to the many and varied side effects of more than 1,000 drugs, I had come across many unique reaction patterns that were reported to be reactions from medications. It had occurred to me that since there is such a proliferation of different prescription and over-the-counter medications, it might be worthwhile to determine which might be responsible for these adverse side effects. Hence this slim manual . . .

I have chosen those medications that have been reported to cause curious, odd, rare, and unique reaction patterns, such as bent penis, eyelash growth, hiccoughs, nightmares, bruxism (grinding teeth), restless legs syndrome, tinnitus (ringing in ears), hallucinations, yawning, compulsive shopping, and the like, as well as a few of the common different bodily responses to drugs; such as itching, hair loss, hives, acne, psoriasis, and lupus. I have described sixty-two of these side effects and the drugs—trade/brand and generic names—that have been reported to trigger them.

There are literally scores of drugs that can provoke all types of reaction patterns, and I have endeavored to mention the most culpable of these. In doing so, and as a function of space constraints, I have intentionally omitted many (not all) of the obscure "chemo" drugs, most of the oral contraceptives, virtually all the medications employed to treat AIDS and HIV infections, as well as the anesthetics utilized during hospital surgical procedures. I have briefly touched on the so-called "biologics" that are employed in the management cases of intractable psoriasis. While topical (surface) medications such as creams, ointments, lotions, and the like can cause reactions on parts of the body other than the skin—for example, people using creams and ointments containing sulfa on the skin can provoke serious, generalized reactions elsewhere—I have included only a few limited references to these.

From the "Top 200 Drugs" list, I have chosen the most commonly employed trade/brand-name prescription and over-the-counter drugs responsible for these reactions. There are literally thousands of these trade/brand-name products, and it would be virtually impossible to list all. Meanwhile the chances are that you have been or are taking at least one of the medications listed in this book.

Who, for example, does not take aspirin? Tylenol? Advil or Motrin? Who is not treated with an antibiotic when suffering from some bacterial or viral infection? How many of you are being medicated with a beta-blocker? An ACE-inhibitor perhaps? Prilosec or Nexium? An antidepressant or sedative? A cholesterol-lowering drug such as Lipitor or Zocor? A nonsteroidal anti-inflammatory drug for arthritis or aches and pains? There is not a medication in the marketplace that cannot give rise to some form of drug reaction in certain hapless sensitive souls.

The incidence of drug reactions increases with age. The likelihood of an adverse drug reaction is three times greater for older persons than for younger adults, and 40 percent of people who suffer an adverse reaction are over age sixty.

It has been documented that more than 100,000 hospitalized patients die from some adverse drug reaction every year. Nearly three billion prescriptions are filled each year; more than 300,000 different over-the-counter medicines are also available; and more than $80 billion are spent each year as a result of drug reactions attributable to these medications.

The most common form of drug reaction on the skin is a measleslike form of rash called an exanthem. Exanthems can be a result of a myriad number of drugs, primarily aspirin, penicillin and its derivatives such as ampicillin and amoxicillin, and a host of other antibacterial agents such as sulfa drugs. Almost one-quarter of all drug reactions on the skin are the result of these antibacterial agents. It is not common knowledge that those people who are allergic to sulfa drugs may also be allergic to medications prescribed for high blood pressure, almost all of which contain some form of thiazide. Thiazide drugs are sulfas! And almost all oral antidiabetic medications are sulfa-based as well. Moreover, many everyday products are sulfa-based. Most sweeteners are sulfa drugs, so if you are allergic to sulfa, you might break out in a rash from sweeteners containing saccharin or cyclamates. (Not, however, aspartame, which is a constituent of Equal and Nutrasweet.) There are also many acne medications, vaginal creams, burn medicines, and eyedrops (Cosopt, Trusopt) that are sulfa-based. Celebrex, used for painful arthritis, is also a sulfa drug. Make sure that your doctor is aware if you are allergic to sulfa drugs (not sulfur, which is an entirely different entity).

Have you been losing hair lately? Perhaps you have been taking a beta-blocker or, if you are a woman, you might be taking hormones such as Provera or other progesterone-containing medication for PMS or for menopausal symptoms. These and other drugs, including Tylenol, Motrin, Advil, birth control pills, antidepressants and tranquilizers, anti-ulcer drugs (Tag-amet and Zantac), can all bring about hair loss, particularly in women. So do many of the "statin" drugs. In addition, al-most all chemotherapeutic agents—drugs employed to treat cancers—can trigger hair loss, reversible in most instances, in both men and women.

Muscle pains and aches have also been reported from tak-ing any of the "statins"—the cholesterol-lowering medications such as Lipitor, Pravachol, Zocor, Mevacor, and others. The "floxin" drugs, such as Cipro and Levaquin, have also been reported to cause severe muscular aches and pains.

Many drugs cause metallic taste, dry mouth, itching, swol-len gums, depression, ringing in the ears, and dozens of other symptoms.

If you are taking any type of medication and you find you have developed some unusual symptom, check with your physician. It may all be a consequence of the drug you have been taking.

Please understand that there are many synonyms for ge-neric medications; for example, Advil, Motrin, Nuprin, and a host of other over-the-counter analgesics are all the same drug called ibuprofen manufactured and promoted by different manufacturers. Tylenol, Paracetamol, Anacin-3, Panadol, and at least two dozen more products are brand names for acet-aminophen; all are the same.

I have listed what I consider to be the 200 most common trade/brand-name drugs and have added a plus sign (+) to those that indicate that there are other brand-name products with the same generic equivalencey. Bactrin and Septra are the same sulfa drug. Atarax and Vistaril are antihistamines that are indistinguishable from one another.

While I have also limited the number of these drugs to 200, there may be many more that could be responsible for ad-verse reactions such as hair loss, hives, itching, depression, and dry mouth.

It is important to remember that not everyone will develop adverse side effects from any specific drug. While there are more than 200 trade/brand-name drugs that can cause tinnitus (ringing in the ears)—I have listed 55 of the most common ones—it does not mean that if you take the same drug you will develop tinnitus. No one knows why only certain individuals will get hives (welts and itching) from aspirin or penicillin, and when you consider that literally millions of people take aspirin every day, it is often a wonder that more people do not develop hives.

I provide a brief overview of all the sixty-two reaction patterns, a few notable people who have suffered through them, and some trivia.

Enjoy!

Jerome Z. Litt, MD

# TRADE/GENERIC NAME MEDICATIONS THAT CAN TRIGGER CURIOUS REACTION PATTERNS

| Trade | Generic |
|-------|---------|
| Abilify | aripiprazole |
| Aciphex | rabeprazole |
| Actonel | risedronate |
| Adderall | dextroamphetamine |
| Aggrenox | dipyridamole |
| Aldara | imiquimod |
| Aleve | naproxen |
| Allegra | fexofenadine |
| Altace | ramipril |
| Ambien | zolpidem |
| Amoxil | amoxicillin |
| Anafranil | clomipramine |
| Androgel | testosterone |
| Antivert | meclizine |
| Aricept | donepezil |
| Asacol | mesalamine |
| Aspirin | dozens of aspirins |
| Astelin | azelastine |
| Atacand | candesartan |
| Atarax | hydoxyzine |
| Ativan | lorazepam |
| Augmentin | amoxicillin |
| Avapro | irbesartan |
| Avelox | moxifloxacin |
| Avodart | dutasteride |
| Axert | almotriptan |
| Axid | nizatidine |
| Bactrim | sulfamethoxazole+ |
| Benicar | olmesartan |
| Biaxin | clarithromycin |
| Botox | Botulinum toxin |
| Buspar | buspirone |
| Cardizem | diltiazem |

| Trade | Generic |
|-------|---------|
| Cardura | doxazosin |
| Casodex | bicalutamide[1] |
| Catapres | clonidine |
| Celebrex | celecoxib |
| Celexa | citalopram |
| CellCept | mycophenolate[2] |
| Chantix | varenicline |
| Cialis | tadalafil |
| Claritin | loratadine |
| Cocaine | cocaine |
| Concerta | methylphenidate |
| Copaxone | glatiramer |
| Coreg | carvedilol |
| Cosopt | dorzolamide+ |
| Coumadin | warfarin |
| Cozaar | losartan |
| Crestor | rosuvastatin |
| Cymbalta | duloxetine |
| Darvocet | propoxyphene+ |
| Depakene | valproic acid |
| Depakote | valproic acid |
| Desyrel | trazodone |
| Detrol | tolterodine |
| Dilantin | phenytoin |
| Diovan | valsartan |
| Ditropan | oxybutynin |
| Duragesic | fentanyl |
| Ecstacy | MDMA |
| Effexor | venlafaxine |
| Elavil | amitriptyline |
| Eldepryl | selegiline |
| Erythromycin | many |
| Evista | raloxifene |
| Exelon | rivastigmine |
| Famvir | famciclovir |
| Femara | letrozole[3] |
| Flexeril | cyclobenzaprine |
| Flomax | tamsulosin |

| Trade | Generic |
| --- | --- |
| Flovent | fluticasone |
| Forteo | teriparatide |
| Fosamax | alendronate |
| Fuzeon | enfuvirtide[4] |
| Geodon | ziprasidone |
| Gleevec | imatinib[5] |
| Glucophage | metformin |
| Haldol | haloperidol |
| hydrochlorothiazide | dozens |
| Humira | adalimumab |
| Hyzaar | losartan+ |
| Imitrex | sumatriptan |
| Inderal | propranolol |
| Indocin | indomethacin |
| Keppra | levetiracetam |
| Klonopin | clonazepam |
| Lamictal | lamotrigine |
| Lamisil | terbinafine |
| Lanoxin | digoxin |
| Lasix | furosemide |
| Levaquin | levofloxacin |
| Levitra | vardenafil |
| Levsinex | hyoscyamine |
| Lexapro | escitalopram |
| Lipitor | atorvastatin |
| Lithobid | lithium |
| Lopid | gemfibrozil |
| Lopressor | metoprolol |
| Lotrel | amlodipine+ |
| Lovenox | enoxaparin |
| Lunesta | eszopiclone |
| Lupron | leuprolide[6] |
| Luvox | fluvoxamine |
| Lyrica | pregabalin |
| Marplan | isocarboxazid |
| Matulane | procarbazine[7] |
| Maxalt | rizatriptan |
| Meridia | sibutramine |

| Trade | Generic |
|-------|---------|
| Micardis | telmisartan+ |
| Minipress | prazosin |
| Minocin | minocycline |
| Mirapex | pramipexole |
| Morphine | many |
| Motrin | ibuprofen |
| MS Contin | morphine |
| Myleran | busulfan[8] |
| Nalfon | fenoprofen |
| Namenda | memantine |
| Nardil | phenelzine |
| Nasonex | mometasone |
| Navane | thiothixene |
| Neurontin | gabapentin |
| Neoral | cyclosporine |
| Nexium | esomeprazole |
| Niaspan | niacin |
| Nicotine | many |
| Nizoral | ketoconazole |
| Norpace | disopyramide |
| Norvasc | amlodipine |
| Oral contraceptives | dozens of OCs |
| OxyContin | oxycodone |
| Pamelor | nortriptyline |
| Parlodel | bromocriptine |
| Paxil | paroxetine |
| Plavix | clopidogrel |
| Pravachol | pravastatin |
| Prevacid | lansoprazole |
| Prilosec | omeprazole |
| Procardia | nifedipine |
| Procrit | epoetin alfa |
| Prograf | tacrolimus |
| Protonix | pantoprazole |
| Provigil | modafinil |
| Prozac | fluoxetine |
| Reglan | metoclopramide |
| Relpax | eletriptan |

| Trade | Generic |
|-------|---------|
| Requip | ropinirole |
| Rheumatrex | methotrexate |
| Rhinocort | budesonide |
| Risperdal | risperidone |
| Ritalin | methylphenidate |
| Rozerem | ramelteon |
| Septra | sulfamethoxazole+ |
| Seroquel | quetiapine |
| Sinemet | levodopa |
| Singulair | montelukast |
| Spiriva | tiotropium |
| Strattera | atomoxetine |
| Suboxone | naloxone+ |
| Synthroid | levothyroxine |
| Tagamet | cimetidine |
| Tegretol | carbamazepine |
| Tenormin | atenolol |
| Thalomid | thalidomide |
| Thorazine | chlorpromazine |
| Timoptic | timolol |
| Toprol | metoprolol |
| Travatan | travaprost |
| Tricor | fenofibrate |
| Trileptal | oxcarbazepine |
| Trizivir | 3 AIDS drugs |
| Tylenol | acetaminophen |
| Ultram | tramadol |
| Valium | diazepam |
| Vancocin | vancomycin |
| Valtrex | valacyclovir |
| Vasotec | enalapril |
| Verelan | verapamil |
| Vesicare | solifenacin |
| Viagra | sildenafil |
| Vicodin | hydrocodone+ |
| Visken | pindolol |
| Vistaril | hydroxyzine |
| Voltaren | diclofenac |

| Trade | Generic |
|-------|---------|
| Vytorin | ezetimibe+ |
| Wellbutrin | bupropion |
| Xanax | alprazolam |
| Xeloda | capecitabine[9] |
| Xenical | orlistat |
| Xopenex | levalbuterol |
| Zestril | lisinopril |
| Zocor | simvastatin |
| Zoloft | sertraline |
| Zomig | zolmitriptan |
| Zonegran | zonisamide |
| Zyban | bupropion |
| Zyprexa | olanzapine |
| Zyrtec | cetirizine |
| Zyvox | linezolid |

(Note: + after the name means other components in it)
[1] for prostate cancer
[2] for prevention of organ rejection
[3] for breast cancer
[4] for HIV
[5] for leukemia
[6] for prostate cancer
[7] for Hodgkin's disease
[8] for leukemia
[9] for breast cancer

# PART A
# NERVOUS SYSTEM
# REACTIONS

## Chapter 1: Compulsions

Compulsions are irresistible impulses to act, regardless of the logic of the motivation. A compulsion is a repetitious, stereotyped, and often insignificant action, the performance of which is compelled even though the person does not wish to perform the act. Three common compulsions, oftentimes the result of medications, are overeating, gambling, and shopping.

### COMPULSIVE OVEREATING

(Binge Eating)

Binge eating—compulsive overeating—is defined as an addiction to food. The essential features of binge eating disorder (BED) are recurrent out-of-control episodes of consuming abnormally large amounts of food. People suffering from BED commit themselves to frequent episodes of uncontrolled eating, or binging, during which they may feel wildly agitated or out of control. They will eat much more rapidly than is normal and continue to eat even past the point of being uncomfortably full. Some people use food like a drug and turn to the "fridge" when problems start to accumulate. Binging in this way is generally followed by a period of extreme guilt feelings and depression.

(BED is similar to, but distinct from, compulsive overeating but the differences are so minuscule that I have taken the liberty of lumping them together. Chronic overeating is an addiction (compulsion) to eat food, like any other addiction. Binge eating is somewhat different in that it can be "triggered" by a general life condition, specific events, or emotions, which are not always obvious. I will employ both terms interchangeably.)

BED is an official eating disorder in the *DSM-IV (Diagnostic and Statistical Manual of Mental Disorders),* a publication of the American Psychiatric Association that classifies more than 200 mental conditions. Although BED has only recently been recognized as a distinct condition, it is probably the most common eating disorder. Most people with binge eating disorder are obese (more than 20 percent above a healthy body weight) and BED is more common in women, with three women affected for every two men. Anger, worry, sorrow, boredom, or other negative emotions can trigger a binge episode.

BED shares some of its attributes with bulimia; the essential difference, however, is that compulsive eaters, while binging out of control, do not attempt to compensate for their binging with purging behavior such as fasting, laxative use or vomiting. Compulsive overeaters will customarily eat when they are not hungry, spend an inordinate amount of time and thoughts dedicated to food, and furtively scheme or fantasize about eating alone.

Compulsive overeaters frequently engage in grazing behavior, during which they return to pick at food continually throughout the day. This can give rise to diabetes, heart disease, high blood pressure, kidney disease, arthritis, bone collapse, high cholesterol, stroke, and depression.

Often beginning in childhood, when eating patterns are taking form, some compulsive overeaters do not learn effective ways of adapting to stress or traumatic situations, so they turn to food in an attempt to control these agonizing feelings. During binges, compulsive overeaters may devour from 5,000 to 60,000 calories per day, precipitating an addictive "high" similar to that which takes place in the course of drug use—a release from psychological stress. Overeating is generally caused by a low self-esteem, the food acting as a substitute for something we feel is wanting in our lives.

## Triggers:
- Being alone, isolated, workaholic lifestyle, lack of structure in the day
- Dieting, breaking a diet, feeling hungry, drinking alcohol
- Involvement in important, non-nurturing relationships that cause low self-worth and stress
- Personal problems (splitting up with a partner, death of a loved one, losing a job)
- Unpleasant feelings—anxiety, frustration, boredom, tiredness, upset, depression, feeling abandoned, anger

BED subjects show the following symptoms:
- Failure to exercise restraint over consumption of food
- Eating between and beyond mealtimes, snacking inordinately
- Eating in secret or alone; feeling humiliated about binging behavior; hiding binging behavior so that even close friends and family members don't know they binge eat
- Eating much more rapidly than ordinarily, and experiencing an "altered state of consciousness"

(trance-like); watching TV or listening to loud music to distract them during binges
- Eating to feel temporary emotional comfort; driven to eat for pleasurable feelings
- Eating abnormally large amounts of food, to the point of feeling physical discomfort
- Eating large amounts of food even when not hungry
- Feeling a sense of being "out of control" while eating; taking other people's food, stealing, eating discarded food, and/or searching desperately for food
- Feeling agitated, wandering and pacing up and down during binges
- Feeling distress, depression, shame, revulsion or disgust after overeating
- Intense desire or cravings to eat particular foods
- Low self-esteem/self-image over concern about shape and weight; trying to diet due to guilt

The major complications of BED include the following:
- Eating foods that are high in sugar and/or salt
- Illnesses as a result of a lack of proper nutrition
- Inability to control BED for very long; skipping work, school, or social activities to binge eat
- Combined with obesity, risk for type 2 diabetes, high blood pressure, high cholesterol, gallbladder disease, heart disease, and certain types of cancer
- High risk of substance-related disorders and serious psychiatric conditions, including depression, panic disorders, anxiety, and personality disorders

## Trivia:

Marlon Brando was a compulsive eater. His eating binges grew to assume legendary proportions. Brando often devoured two whole chickens, half a cheesecake, and a pint of ice cream in a single sitting. He was also famous for driving to a food stand in the very early morning to stuff himself on several hot dogs. He was famous for eating boxes of Mallomars and cinnamon buns and washing them down with a quart of milk. During the shooting of *One-Eyed Jacks* (1961), he would have "two steaks, potatoes, two apple pies á la mode and a quart of milk" for dinner, entailing endless altering of his costumes. His second wife, Movita, recounted times when he drove down to hot dog stands late at night, scarfing down as many as six at a time. *Mutiny on the Bounty* (1962) costumer James Taylor claimed that Brando split the seat on fifty-two pairs of pants during the shooting of the film, necessitating that stretch fabric be sewn into Marlon's replacement togs. He split those, too.

Medications that have been known to cause binge eating include the following:

## Trade/Brand-names

| | | |
|---|---|---|
| Ambien | Levsinex | Seroquel |
| Betapace | Lipitor | Sonata |
| Botox | Lunesta | Sustiva |
| Dalmane | Migranal | Topamax |
| Ditropan | Niaspan | Tylenol |
| Dolophine | Orinase | Ultracet |
| Doral | Parlodel | Ultram |
| Duragesic | Prevacid | Vfend |
| Ecstacy | ProSom | Viread |
| Glucophage | Restoril | Zyrtec |
| Halcion | Rozerem | |
| Indocin | Seconal | |

## COMPULSIVE GAMBLING

(Pathologic Gambling; Ludopathy)

> Whatever Voltaire or Descartes may say—
> The world for me is a pack of cards,
> Life is the bank; fate deals, I play
> And the rules of the game I apply to people.
> —Russian poet Mikhail Lermontov (1814–1841)

Compulsive or pathologic gambling, a chronic and progressive mental illness, is an impulse-control disorder. This addiction is marked by a dogged inability to resist the temptation to gamble. Compulsive gamblers tend to lose control of the amounts they risk and are incapable of putting a stop to their gambling even when they continue to lose. Affecting their personal, social and work life, this serious psychiatric disorder leads to significant anguish and stress to those afflicted, their families, and their friends. The number of existing cases of compulsive gambling in the United States has increased with that of gambling itself, and it is estimated that up to 3 percent of the adult population gambles obsessively.

To qualify as dysfunctional gambling; the activity must meet at least five of the following criteria:
- Bailout: the person appeals to family and friends for financial help.
- Chasing one's losings: the individual tries to win back losses with more gambling.
- Escape: the subject gambles to circumvent problems.
- Illegal acts: the person breaks the law—theft, forgery, fraud, scams, embezzlement—in order to recover gambling losses.
- Loss of discipline: the person has failed his or her efforts to reduce gambling.

- Lying: the person tries to conceal gambling by lying to family, friends, and therapists.
- Preoccupation: being obsessed with gambling, reliving past gambling experiences, and cooking up ways to get money with which to gamble.
- Risking significant relationships: the person gambles despite jeopardizing a personal relationship or job.
- Tolerance: the subject demands larger or more frequent wagers to recapture the same sudden brief exhilaration.
- Withdrawal: jitteriness or crabbiness related to efforts to end gambling.

Gambling has existed since ancient times, and there is proof that most cultures sanctioned it in one form or another. Paraphernalia linked with gambling have been found in ancient sites in China dating back to 2300 BCE. Ivory dice made before 1500 BCE have been found in Egypt and writings alluding to gambling have been discovered on a tablet in one of the pyramids at Giza. Citizens of ancient India, Greece, and Rome also did their share of gambling.

Gambling was so popular during the Middle Ages that some militaries prohibited their soldiers from taking part in games, as the gambling interfered with their assigned responsibilities.

Islam, consistently condemns gambling; in Islamic societies gambling is either totally forbidden or very restricted. The Koran explicitly denounces gambling as sinful.

Christianity has always been critical of gambling (Matt. 6: 25–26; Luke 12:15; Hebrews 13:5). Early Church councils forbade games of chance, and up to the time of the Reformation (sixteenth century) the Church in general viewed gambling as sinful and deplorable. Lutheran churches have been harsh in their condemnation of gambling.

One of the most famous addicted gamblers was John Montagu, the Earl of Sandwich. In 1762, he sat for over twenty-four hours at a gaming table in his home, declining to attend meals. Eventually, one of his servants offered the Earl a piece of salted beef. The Earl ordered the servant to put the beef between two slices of bread so that he could eat it in his hand while at the table. This is how the sandwich got its name.

*The Gambler*, one of the most psychologically profound and successful of Fyodor Dostoevsky's works, is a good case history of a compulsive gambler in literature. Based on the author's addiction to gambling, the novel is widely regarded as autobiographical.

Tchaikovsky's opera, *The Queen of Spades*, based on Alexander Pushkin's short story about human avariciousness, is the story of a Russian engineer who becomes obsessed with the secret of three consecutive winning cards after hearing a story about an old countess's winnings several years before. The subject of the opera is, for the most part, the destructive and isolating nature of gambling addiction.

Imbalances in the brain chemicals: serotonin, norepinephrine (adrenaline), and dopamine may be factors in compulsive gambling. Serotonin plays a key role in regulating mood and behavior. Norepinephrine, a hormone released in response to stress, has been linked to arousal and risk-taking in compulsive gamblers.

There is a credible link between pathological gambling and the drugs that raise the level of dopamine in the brain. Dopamine, a chemical neurotransmitter essential to the normal functioning of the central nervous system, plays a crucial role in the way the brain controls movements. Brain cells release dopamine as part of the reward system through which one learns to seek pleasurable stimuli, such as food and sex, and dopamine plays a role in developing addiction. A reduced concentration of dopamine within the brain is also associated with Parkinsonism.

Patients with Parkinsonism who take certain antitremor medications are at greater risk of becoming pathological gamblers. These antitremor drugs, known as dopamine agonists, are also associated with other addictive behaviors such as compulsive shopping, binge eating, punding (hobbyism), drug use, and other pleasurable experiences such as alcohol intake and sex. These are linked by their reward-seeking or incentive-based and repetitious natures.

Medications that have been associated with compulsive gambling include the following:

<u>Trade/Brand-names</u>

| | | |
|---|---|---|
| Alcohol | Intropin | Parlodel |
| Dostinex | Mirapex | Requip |
| Haldol | Neopro | Sinemet |

## COMPULSIVE SHOPPING

(Oniomania)

> Anybody who says money can't buy you
> happiness doesn't know where to shop
> —Joan Collins

Compulsive buying disorder—sometimes called compulsive shopping disorder or oniomania—is defined as an undisciplined zest to acquire all kinds of things, especially the unessential and the unaffordable. It is common for those afflicted to go on repeated shopping binges and then to amass large quantities of unnecessary, unneeded, and unwanted items. This repetitive, excessive, and inappropriate buying produces an emotional high in compulsive shoppers, followed by a sense of guilt when they recognize how much they have spent.

Oniomania (from Greek *onios* meaning "for sale," coined by German psychiatrist Emil Kraepelin,) also known as shopping addiction or shopaholism, is the compulsive desire to shop. For those addicted to shopping, buying for the sake of buying generates a feeling of satisfaction, seems to give their life a meaning, and enables them to forget their sorrows.

Compulsive shoppers often shop when they feel depressed, lonely, bored, or angry. This "hidden epidemic" occurs mainly in developed countries where the availability of a wide variety of goods, easily gotten credit, disposable income, and significant leisure time are common. This compulsion offers those who suffer from it a compensation for their pain and suffering, and they believe that shopping will make them feel better. Compulsive shoppers often show a great fashion sense and have an intense interest in new clothing styles and products.

Shopping may occur in just about any environment or surrounding, ranging from high-end department stores and boutiques to consignment shops or garage sales. Among women, favorite categories for items purchased by compulsive shoppers include clothing, shoes, jewelry, makeup, and music. Men tend to have a greater preference than women for electronic, automotive, and hardware merchandise.

According to the American Psychological Association, there are more than 15 million "oniomaniacs" in the United States. Between 80 to 95 percent of those affected are female. Men are often characterized as "collectors" and women as shopaholics. Onset usually occurs in the late teens or early twenties, the disorder is generally chronic, and the outcomes can include bankruptcy, divorce, embezzlement, and occasionally suicide attempts.

Oniomania is one of the impulse control disorders (ICDs), a group of relatively common psychiatric conditions. ICDs, which are listed in the *DSM,* typically involve pleasurable behaviors (gambling, shopping, or sex) that are performed repetitively, excessively, or compulsively to an extent that interferes in normal life functioning. Some researchers have compared compulsive buying to addictive disorders, like alcohol and drug use; some have considered it an obsessive-compulsive disorder (OCD); and others classify it as a mood disorder.

Behaviors typical of compulsive shopping and spending include any or all of the following:

- Buying items on credit, via catalogs, "home shopping networks," or on the Internet, that would not be bought with cash
- Feeling a rush of elation, joy, and anxiety when spending money
- Feeling guilty, ashamed, embarrassed, or confused after shopping or spending extravagantly
- Feeling lost without credit cards
- Arguing with others about one's shopping or spending habits
- Lying to others about purchases made or how much money had been spent
- Shopping for the sheer excitement of the buying itself and the accompanying thrill of bargain hunting
- Shopping or spending habits causing emotional suffering in one's life
- Shopping or spending money as a result of feeling disappointed, angry, or worried
- Spending a lot of time juggling accounts or bills to adjust to spending
- Thinking excessively about money

Women shopaholics tend to consider their purchases as opportunities not to be neglected and they often exhibit the following characteristics:

- Their links to online shopping sites are longer and more frequent.
- They consider their purchases as personally fulfilling.
- They have a higher tendency to use items less often than they had expected.
- They more often make purchases to impress others.
- They spend appreciably more time speaking on their cell phones.

One example of shopaholism is the case of Antoinette Millard. Millard, the daughter of a steelworker, passed herself off in Manhattan as a Saudi princess who had converted to Judaism. Millard purchased jewels as though they were bonbons, and mixed with New York's fashionable elite. In three months, she spent over one million dollars on her no-limit American Express Centurion card. On May 8, 2004, Millard became the focus of media attention in New York when she claimed that she had been mugged and robbed of her insured jewelry worth a quarter of a million dollars. Having insured her purchases, she then reported them stolen, hoping to cash in on the insurance proceeds. Millard was arrested and committed to a mental institution for her unmanageable and refractory shopping addiction.

Notable people who are or have been compulsive shoppers include the following:

- Imelda Marcos of the Philippines was the quintessential shopaholic, although she could be better described as a "shoeaholic." After the Marcos family fled Malacañang Palace, Imelda was found to own 15 mink coats, 508 gowns, 888 handbags, 300 bras (one of which was bulletproof), and 1,060 pairs of shoes.
- Elton John, famous for his legendary spending sprees, reportedly spent $850,000 on a single day. He once spent $200,000 on flowers. Asked why, he replied, "Well, I like flowers."
- Marie Antoinette's spending orgies incited the fury that provoked the French Revolution.
- Mary Todd Lincoln spent more on clothes than any other First Lady. She bought 300 pairs of lace gloves in four months, leaving the Lincoln family in enormous debt.
- William Randolph Hearst was a legendary collector of art and antiques.

- Jacqueline Kennedy Onassis had a serious clothing addiction.
- Princess Diana was also notorious for her clothing addiction.
- Britney Spears, with an estimated $200 million in the bank, shops when she's depressed.
- Victoria Beckham, a former Spice Girl, is believed to spend $200,000 a year on her wardrobe, and has turned shopping into her main occupation. "I can't help it," she says. "When I see something I like, I buy it in every color and I buy shoes in every color to match, as well as handbags. If I could, I'd go shopping every single day. I'm definitely a shopaholic."

In rare cases dopamine agonists, which are being used in the treatment of disorders such as Parkinsonism and restless legs syndrome, can cause compulsive behavior, such as an uncontrollable desire to shop. Some of these medications include the following:

### Trade/Brand-names

| | | |
|---|---|---|
| Ambien | Mirapex | Permax |
| Apokyn | Neupro | Requip |
| Dostinex | Parlodel | |

# Chapter 2: Erectile Dysfunction (ED) and Penile Disorders

## Erectile Dysfunction (ED); (Impotence)

Erectile dysfunction—also known as impotence—is the term used to describe the inability of a male to attain and maintain an erect penis that is rigid enough to permit satisfactory sexual intercourse.

ED, as it is known, has been estimated to affect about 20 million men in the United States and countless millions throughout the world. The incidence of this problem increases with age. In the United States, less than 1 percent of the male population under thrity years of age is affected, 3 percent under forty-five years, 7 percent between forty-five and fifty-five years, 25 percent at age sixty-five, and up to 75 percent in men eighty years old. A recent study estimated that more than 150 million men worldwide experience some degree of impotence. In addition, based on population projections, it is likely that the prevalence of the condition will more than double over the next twenty-five years.

Impotence may result from psychological, neurologic, hormonal, or physical impairment or it may be a result of a combination of these factors. Other than disease, the most common psychological factors contributing to impotence are stress in a man's life or difficulties in his sexual and personal relationships. Many impotent men have been affected initially by a purely physical problem, but by the time they seek treatment, their condition is complicated by psychological factors. Augmented by anxiety, depression, and low self-esteem, this disorder can be disastrous.

Excessive alcohol use has long been recognized as one cause of impotence, leading to the euphemism "brewer's droop" or "whiskey dick"; Shakespeare made light of this phenomenon in *Macbeth*.

Causes of impotence are related to physical conditions, disease, trauma, psychological factors, and medications, and include the following:

- Aging
- Cigarette smoking
- Depression
- Diabetes (in 40 percent of the cases in the United States)
- Endocrine (glandular) problems
- Kidney failure and dialysis
- Liver disease
- Low testosterone levels
- Medications (see below)
- Multiple sclerosis
- Spinal cord injury
- Surgery on the pelvis or penis
- Vascular diseases

The oldest reference to impotence was made in the Sushruta Samhita, around the eighth century BCE in India. The ancient Hindus believed that impotence could be of mental origin, from intercourse with a distasteful woman.

The ancient Egyptian papyrus Ebers, a medical document dated 1600 BCE, recommended baby crocodiles' hearts mixed with wood oil to be smeared into the husband's penis to restore his potency.

The word impotence is derived from the Latin word *impotencia*, which literally translated means lack of power. The first recorded use of the word impotence to mean loss of sexual power was in 1655.

Impotence, often considered to be caused by a divine curse, was mentioned in the Old Testament. King Abimelech is believed to have become impotent as punishment for taking Abraham's wife, Sarah, who was introduced to him as Abraham's sister: *But God came to Abimelech in a dream by night and said to him: Behold, thou art but a dead man, for the woman which thou has taken for she is a man's wife* (Genesis 20:3).

One famous case involved Don Carlos II, the last of the Spanish Hapsburg kings, who was unable to provide a Spanish heir through presumed impotence. Thus, the issue of the inheritance of the Spanish kingdoms—which included not only Spain, but Italy, the Low Countries, and the Americas—became quite contentious. This eventually led to the War of Spanish Succession (1701–1714).

"If a woman's hand, which is the best of all remedies, is not good enough to cure the flabbiness of a man's penis, the other remedies will do little." Unfortunately, this quote by the Frenchman Nicholas Vennette (1633–1698) summed up the casual and generally held view by both the public and the medical profession about impotence and its treatments.

Normally, when a man becomes sexually aroused, his penis increases in size, becoming erect and rigid, enabling sexual penetration. An average penis is between three inches and four inches long; when it is erect it increases in length to between five and seven inches. An erection occurs when the penis fills with blood. An erect penis contains six or seven times the blood volume of a flaccid penis. As an aside, and to dispel a few myths, penis size has little or no relation to sexual pleasure or performance.

The medicines listed below have been reported to produce ED as a side effect:

## Trade/Brand-names

| | | |
|---|---|---|
| Abilify | Haldol | Percodan |
| Aldactone | Inderal | Phenergan |
| Aldomet | Lanoxin | Pravachol |
| Aleve | Lasix | Prexige |
| Amicar | Librium | Procardia |
| Anafranil | Lipitor | Prolixin |
| Antivert | Lithobid | Propecia |
| Apresoline | Loniten | Proscar |
| Ativan | Lopid | Prozac |
| Axid | Lopressor | Regitine |
| Bumex | Lupron | Reglan |
| Buspar | Marplan | Serax |
| Calan | Maxzide | Serentil |
| Capoten | Mellaril | Serpasil |
| Casodex | Mevacor | Sinemet |
| Catapres | Micardis | Sinequan |
| Celebrex | Minipress | Stelazine |
| Chantix | Morphine | Tagamet |
| Cocaine | Myleran | Tenex |
| Compazine | Nardil | Tenormin |
| Cordarone | Navane | Thalidomid |
| Cymbalta | Nebilet | Thorazine |
| Demerol | Nicoderm | Tofranil |
| Desyrel | Nicotine | Tranxene |
| Dilantin | Nizoral | Valium |
| Dilaudid | Norflex | Vasotec |
| Diovan | Normodyne | Verelan |
| Diuril | Norpace | Vistaril |
| Dolophine | Norpramin | Wytensin |
| Duragesic | Norvasc | Yohimbine |
| Elavil | OxyContin | Zantac |
| Eskalith | Pamelor | Zocor |
| Estrogen | Parlodel | Zoloft |
| Eulexin | Parnate | |
| Flexeril | Pepcid | |

## Peyronie's Disease

### (Bent Penis or "Bent Nail" Syndrome)

Peyronie's disease—not really a disease—is a connective tissue disorder involving the growth of fibrous plaques—essentially patches of thickened fibers—in the soft tissue of the penis. Affecting about 1–4 percent of men, it is associated with an uncharacteristic curvature of the penis—bent penis—when erect. It primarily affects Caucasian men between forty-five and sixty years of age. Because of unwillingness to seek medical attention for the condition and failure to report cases with mild symptoms, the incidence may be higher. It is not cancerous.

Erectile dysfunction often occurs with this curvature in the later stages of the disease process, and narrowing or shortening of the penis, as well as pain, may materialize. Peyronie's disease, bearing the name of a Frenchman, Francois de la Peyronie, can be a physically and psychologically disquieting disorder. At times, pain, bending, and emotional distress make sexual intercourse virtually impossible. For many men with Peyronie's disease, the malady never goes beyond the inflammation stage, which more often than not resolves without treatment within a year or so.

About 30 percent of men with Peyronie's disease develop fibrosis in other elastic tissues of the body, such as on the hand (Dupuytren's contracture) or foot.

Awareness of Peyronie's disease grew when President Bill Clinton's erect penis was revealed as having an angled bend visible during a sexual misconduct case.

In 1587, an anatomist, Giulio Cesare Aranzi, described an unusual curvature of the penis in the medical literature of his day. Aranzi and other physicians, surgeons, pathologists, and anatomists had observed and described penile curvature prior to Peyronie, who described three cases in 1743. As surgeon to King Louis XV, he was already a celebrity, and so he garnered the glory.

Medications that have been reported to trigger Peyronie's disease include the following:

### Trade/Brand-names

| | | |
|---|---|---|
| Alprostadil | Rheumatrex | Trandate |
| Col-Benemid | Timoptic | |
| Cosopt | Toprol | |

## Priapism

(Painful Erection)

Priapism is a prolonged and usually painful erection of the penis resulting from either a medical condition or medications. Lasting up to several hours to several days, it is not associated with sexual thoughts or sexual activity. When it occurs in women, it is known as clitorism.

Sickle-cell anemia, leukemia, and spinal cord injury are probably the most common medical conditions that cause priapism. It is a urologic emergency, and a urologic consultation should be obtained as early as possible.

In Greek mythology, Priapus, a Phrygian fertility and virility god, was the son of Aphrodite and Dionysius. He was best noted for his enormous, permanently erect penis, which gave rise to the medical term priapism. On account of the reproductive function of his virile member, Priapus has been regarded as the God of procreation—symbolizing the male procreative power. Priapus then became, predictably, the patron of all in need of luck, especially men and women in search of sexual gratification. Equally important was Priapus' power to ward off the evil eye. In those days people often wore the phallic amulet of Priapus and decorated their homes with images of his erect penis. Statues of Priapus were popular in ancient Greek and Roman gardens and doorways, and travelers would caress the statue's penis as they passed by. This fertility statue also served as a scarecrow to fend off birds, animals, and other scavengers.

The mythology of Priapus has two noteworthy tales. In one, Priapus argues with an ass about relative penis size. Priapus wins the contest and then beats the ass to death. In the second, Priapus lusts after the nymph Lotis, the daughter of Poseidon. Priapus tries to rape her as she sleeps, but just as he is about to assault her, an ass alerts her with his braying.

In a case recorded in a German newspaper: "Erection Keeps Burglar Out of Jail": a burglar escaped a prison sentence because he was afflicted with a permanent erection and entered a hospital as an "emergency case" for his persistent priapism. After a week's treatment, doctors admitted they were only able to get his erection down to "half-mast." To the dismay of the police prosecutor, a court ruled that he could stay out of jail while his problem remained.

Well-known movie and TV actor Tom Sizemore, a self-proclaimed sex addict, allegedly suffers from priapism that leaves him aroused for hours. As an actor in a celebrity sex video, this disease may have been the invention of an overzealous public relations department.

A "death erection" or "terminal erection"—technically a priapism and sometimes referred to as "angel lust"—is a postmortem erection that is noted in the corpses of human males who have been executed, particularly by hanging. A postmortem priapism indicates that death was likely swift and violent.

Samuel Beckett's *Waiting for Godot* alludes to priapism in Act I:

> Estragon: What about hanging ourselves?
> Vladimir: Hmm. It'd give us an erection.
> Estragon: (highly excited). An erection!
> Vladimir: With all that follows. Where it falls mandrakes grow. That's why they shriek when you pull them up. Did you not know that?
> Estragon: Let's hang ourselves immediately!

At the end of Herman Melville's novel *Billy Budd*, Billy's unusual moral purity is suggested by the fact that, contrary to the general rule, he does not get an erection after being hanged.

On the other hand, in Thomas Pynchon's novel *Mason & Dixon*, Charles Mason says to himself "In my experience, 'tis usually the Innocent who get terminal erections, and the Guilty who fail to."

In Thomas Harris's third Hannibal Lecter novel, *Hannibal*, the hanging of Inspector Pazzi by Dr. Fell causes a death erection.

Medications that have been reported to induce priapism include the following:

## Trade/Brand-names

| | | |
|---|---|---|
| Abilify | Eskalith | Luvox |
| Android | Flomax | Marihuana |
| Apokyn | Geodon | Marplan |
| Atarax | Haldol | Maxzide |
| Cardura | Heparin | Mellaril |
| Celexa | Hytrin | Mevacor |
| Cialis | Inapsin | Micardis |
| Clopixol | Innohep | Minipress |
| Clozaril | Isoptin | Moban |
| Cocaine | Kemadrin | Morphine |
| Compazine | Lanoxin | Muse |
| Concerta | Lasix | Myleran |
| Copaxone | Lescol | Naprosyn |
| Coumadin | Levitra | Nardil |
| Desyrel | Lexapro | Navane |
| Dilantin | Librium | Nebilet |
| Diprivan | Lipitor | Nicoderm |
| Ecstacy | Lithobid | Nicotine |
| Effexor | Loniten | Nizoral |
| Elavil | Lopid | Norflex |
| Elestat | Lopressor | Normodyne |
| Ephedrie | Lupron | Norpace |

## Trade/Brand-names

| | | |
|---|---|---|
| Norpramin | Reglan | Tofranil |
| Norvasc | Risperdal | Tranxene |
| OxyContin | Ritalin | Trilafon |
| Pamelor | Rogitine | Trileptal |
| Parlodel | Serax | Uroxatral |
| Parnate | Serentil | Valium |
| Pavabid | Seroquel | Vancocin |
| Paxil | Serpasil | Vasotec |
| Pepcid | Serzone | Verelan |
| Percodan | Sinemet | Viagra |
| Phenergan | Sinequan | Vistaril |
| Pravachol | Sporanox | Wellbutrin |
| Prexige | Stelazine | Wytensin |
| Procardia | Strattera | Yohimbine |
| Prograf | Tagamet | Zantac |
| Prolixin | Tenex | Zocor |
| Propecia | Tenormin | Zoloft |
| Proscar | Testoderm | Zyban |
| Prozac | Thalidomid | Zyprexa |
| Regitine | Thorazine | |

# Chapter 3:
# Hallucinations

A hallucination is seeing, hearing, touching, smelling, or tasting something that is not there. It is a sensory perception without a source in the external world. The word "hallucination" comes from the Latin *hallucinari*, meaning "to wander in the mind." Patients suffering from dementia and psychotic disorders such as schizophrenia often experience hallucinations. About 40–50 percent of patients diagnosed with Alzheimer's disease develop hallucinations in the advanced stages of the disease. About 75 percent of adults diagnosed with adult-onset schizophrenia experience hallucinations, most commonly auditory or visual.

In 2000, one of the few studies of hallucinations in a general Western population reported the following: of a total sample of 13,000 adults, 40 percent reported hallucinations: 6 percent had hallucinations once a month, 3 percent once a week, and 2 percent more than once a week.

Hallucinations are rare in children under the age of eight. However, about 40 percent of children diagnosed with schizophrenia have visual or auditory hallucinations.

## Visual Hallucinations

Visual hallucinations are false perceptions of sight, which may include colors, shapes, or flashes of light, but are typically of people or humanlike figures. For example, one may perceive a person standing before him or her when no one is there. About 14 percent of patients treated in eye clinics for glaucoma or age-related macular degeneration report visual hallucinations. Ten percent of patients diagnosed with migraine headaches experience visual hallucinations preceding the on-set of an acute attack.

Visual hallucinations can start with misinterpretations: the person thinks he or she sees faces or objects in spiraling pat-terns on fabrics or in the shadows in a room. Visual hallucina-tions, involving people, animals, insects, convoluted scenes, or weird situations, are the most common type of hallucination in dementia; they are commonly reported by patients receiving treatment for Parkinsonism.

Although classically associated with psychiatric disorders, the hallucinatory experience can be associated with several conditions:

- Alcohol withdrawal syndrome
- Endocrine disorders
- Grief
- Infectious diseases
- Medication reactions (see below)
- Brain injury
- Migraine headaches
- Narcolepsy
- Neurological disorders
- Parkinsonism
- Poor eyesight
- Post-traumatic stress disorder (PTSD)
- Psychosis
- Seizures
- Sleep disorders
- Stress
- Substance abuse
- Temporal lobe epilepsy

Medications that have been reported to cause visual hal-lucinations include the following:

## Trade/Brand-names

Accupril
Akineton
Aldoril
Ambien
Aminophylline
Amoxapine
Amphetamines
Anafranil
Antabuse
Antivert
Azulfidine
Benadryl
Benzodiazepines
Biaxin
Catapres
Cerebyx
Cocaine
Cogentin
Concerta
Cortisone-like drugs
Dantrium
Dapsone
Depakene
Depakote
Desoxyn
Dilantin
Dramamine
Ecstacy
Eldepryl
Ephedra
Inderal
INH
Ismotic
Kemadrin
Ketalar
Lanoxin
Lasix
Lescol

Librium
Lipitor
Lithobid
Loniten
Lopid
Lopressor
LSD
Ludiomil
Lupron
Marihuana
Marplan
Maxzide
Mellaril
Mescaline
Mevacor
Micardis
Minipress
Morphine
Muse
Myleran
Mysoline
Naprosyn
Nardil
Navane
Nebilet
Nicoderm
Nicotine
Nizoral
Norflex
Normodyne
Norpace
Norpramin
Norvasc
OxyContin
Pamelor
Parlodel
Parnate
Penetrex

Pepcid
Percodan
Phenergan
Phenobarbital
Phenylpropa-
   nolamine
Placidyl
Platinol
Pravachol
Prexige
Procardia
Prolixin
Pronestyl
Propecia
Proscar
Prozac
Regitine
Reglan
Ritalin
Robitussin
Rynatuss
Serax
Serentil
Serpasil
Sinemet
Sinequan
Stelazine
Symmetrel
Tagamet
Tambocor
Tenex
Tenormin
Tetracyclines
Thalidomid
Thorazine
Tofranil
Tonocard
Tranxene

<u>Trade/Brand-names</u>

| | | |
|---|---|---|
| Valium | Viagra | Zanaflex |
| Valtrex | Vincasar | Zantac |
| Vasotec | Vistaril | Zarontin |
| Verelan | Wytensin | Zocor |
| Vfend | Yohimbine | Zoloft |

## Auditory Hallucinations

Auditory hallucinations, the false or distorted perceptions of sound, music, noises, or voices "are one of the most terrifying, and ill-understood tricks the human psyche is capable of." Hearing voices when there is no auditory trigger is the most common type of auditory hallucination in mental disorders. In schizophrenia, a frequent symptom is to hear voices conversing. Auditory hallucinations can range from rudimentary sounds to speech and music. These are some of the most awe-inspiring manifestations experienced by the mentally ill. The perception of these sounds or voices can be very frightening, can occur at any time, and are very difficult to treat. The voices may instruct the person to perform an act (commonly referred to as "command hallucinations"). The man who killed a Swedish politician in September 2003 told the police that voices in his head told him "to attack." Studies of combat veterans diagnosed with post-traumatic stress disorder (PTSD) have found that 50 to 65 percent have encountered auditory hallucinations.

Auditory hallucinations are most often a symptom of severe, incapacitating psychiatric or neurological illness. They affect about 70 percent of those with schizophrenia and about 15 percent of those with mood disorders such as depression or psychosis.

True auditory hallucinations occur when people distinctly hear voices or other noises despite the fact that nothing is there. These voices can produce an outpouring of speech, often obscene or derogatory, or a running commentary on one's private views and opinions. Musical hallucinations, where people hear familiar music playing in their mind, is a type of auditory hallucination. This can be caused by lesions on the brain, often occurring from strokes, but also from tumors, encephalitis, or abscesses.

Musical hallucinations, most common in older people, especially women with hearing loss, can result from listening to music for long periods of time. Beethoven had musical hallucinations after he became deaf.

Auditory hallucinations have been described in conjunction with many situations and diseases, including the following:
- Bereavement
- Brain abscesses
- Brain tumors
- Drug poisoning
- Encephalitis
- Near-death experiences
- Psychiatric or neurological disorders
- Religious phenomena
- Strokes

Many historical figures—Socrates, Caesar, Descartes—have been reported to "hear voices." Hallucinated voices are also known to occur during states of religious or creative inspiration. Joan of Arc described hearing the voices of saints telling her to free her country from the English. Rainer Maria Rilke heard the voice of a "terrible angel" accompanied by the sound of a crashing sea after living alone in a castle on the Adriatic for two months. This experience prompted his writing the poem, *Duino Elegies*.

Absinthe, a bitter spirit containing wormwood, was one of the most popular alcoholic beverages of late nineteenth-century Europe. The emerald green drink—"the green fairy"—was consumed by people from all walks of life. Side effects from the active ingredient—thujone—include hallucinations, seizures, and death. The most memorable celebrity known as an absinthe drinker was Vincent van Gogh. Henri de Toulouse-Lautrec, Paul Gauguin, Oscar Wilde, and Edgar Allan Poe were all passionate about absinthe.

The following medical conditions are some of the possible causes of auditory hallucinations:
- Alcohol withdrawal
- Delirium
- Dementia
- Depression
- Drug use (see below)
- Narcolepsy
- Neurological disorders
- Schizophrenia
- Sleep deprivation
- Temporal lobe epilepsy

The following medications have been reported to give rise to auditory hallucinations:

### Trade/Brand-names

| | | |
|---|---|---|
| Ambien | Demerol | Symmetrel |
| Amphetamines | Ketalar | Ultram |
| Catapres | Neo-Synephrine | Tenuate |
| Celontin | Persantine | Valtrex |
| Darvocet | Prialt | Vioxx |
| Darvon | Provigil | Visken |

## Olfactory Hallucinations

(Parosmia/Phantosmia)

An olfactory hallucination is a false perception of odor or smell. The experience is usually very unpleasant: the stench of decaying fish, sewage, dead bodies, or burning rubber. Two of these perverted senses of smell are parosmia and phantosmia.

## Parosmia

(Distorted Smell)

Parosmia, also called troposmia, parosphresia, and parosphresis, is a perversion or distortion of the sense of smell, often resulting in nonexistent, and mostly unpleasant, smells. It is a disorder of the sense of smell elicited by an odor but incorrectly perceived. The affected person sniffs one odor but smells another—usually an offensive one. The person sniffs a banana but it smells like rotting flesh. About two million people in the United States have parosmia.

The sensation of parosmia has always been reported to be unpleasant, typically described as a foul, rotten, sewage, or burning smell. When a normal person smells an unpleasant scent, sensory adaptation takes place quickly, and within a few minutes that scent seems to fade away. The unpleasant scents in parosmia can severely affect the quality of life and can be long-lasting.

Medications that have been reported to cause parosmia include the following:

### Trade/Brand-names

| | | |
|---|---|---|
| Anafranil | Eldepryl | Prevacid |
| Ansaid | Exovac | Remeron |
| Astelin | Fabrazyme | Sonata |
| Avelox | Flumadine | Tasmar |
| Axert | Iopidine | Zomig |
| Azilect | Lipitor | Zonegran |
| Cardura | Miacalcin | Zyrtec |
| Chantix | Norvasc | |

## Phantosmia

Phantosmia involves olfactory hallucinations—smelling an odor without the presence of an odor source, in essence a phantom smell, usually of something unpleasant. Unexplained unpleasant smells are basic symptoms of this disorder where the smell can be something like rotting flesh, vomit, smoke, fish, feces, or garbage. This condition is generally thought to arise from damage to the nervous tissues in the olfactory system as a result of the following:

- Epilepsy
- Exposure to certain toxins
- Head trauma
- Parkinsonism
- Surgery
- Viral infection

Sometimes the condition is considered psychiatric in origin.

No specific drugs have been implicated as the cause of phantosmia.

## Tactile Hallucinations

(Formication)

Also known as a haptic hallucination, a tactile hallucination is a false perception or sensation of touch or something happening in or on the body. A common tactile hallucination, often occurring in drug users, is feeling as if something is crawling on or under the skin. This is also known as formication (see below). People in delirium tremens (the "DTs") withdrawing from alcohol often have this type of hallucination.

## Formication

> The ant has made himself illustrious
> Through constant industry industrious.
> So what?
> Would you be calm and placid
> If you were full of formic acid?
> —Ogden Nash

Formication, essentially a tactile hallucination, is an abnormal skin sensation similar to that of insects crawling over or within the skin.

The term formication has been in use for several hundred years. The 1797 edition of the Encyclopaedia Britannica describes a condition called *raphania* that includes these symptoms: horrid convulsions of the limbs, preceded by a formication, or sensation as of ants or other small insects creeping on the parts.

From the Latin *formicare,* meaning to creep like an ant, formication was described in 1890 as "a variety of itching, often encountered in the eczema of elderly people. It is described as exactly like the crawling of myriads of animals over the skin. It is probably due to the successive irritation of nerve fibers in the skin. At times, patients who suffer from it will scarcely be persuaded that it is not due to insects. Yielding to the temptation to scratch invariably makes the disease worse."

This illusion or hallucination that ants or other insects are creeping on or under the skin is a frequent side effect of large-scale use of cocaine, amphetamines ("amphetamites"), or crystal meth (also known by street names such as "ice," "glass," "chalk," "crank," "meth mites," or "coke bugs"). Formication is also a common side effect of many prescription drugs such as Ritalin, Adderall, and Lunesta (see below). People suffering from formication, particularly if they are delirious or intoxicated, may pick and scratch themselves to such an extent that they trigger self-induced bleeding and excoriations of the skin on areas easy to reach: the face, scalp, neck, thighs, and forearms. This self-mutilation often leads to gouged out pits and ulcers.

Patients often seek countless opinions from physicians, exterminators, and entomologists, and then often complain about the ineffectiveness of the advice received while regarding the specialist with hostility and suspicion.

Formication has been associated with the following:

• Substance abuse

- Diabetic neuropathy
- Diseases of the spinal cord and peripheral nerves
- Extreme alcohol withdrawal with delirium tremens
- Herpes zoster (shingles)
- Menopause
- Skin cancer

Delusions of parasitosis that are not related to drug abuse are more common among middle-aged and elderly women. Patients with this disorder may be fully functional yet have a false belief that they are infested with parasites. They may claim to have the parasites in a collection of material (typically pieces of skin, scabs, hair, lint, dried blood, flies or ants, and other debris) and request that it be examined under a microscope or sent to the laboratory for verification. This clinical presentation is called the "matchbox sign" because patients have often used a matchbox to collect the material. Now small plastic bags—Baggies—are commonly used for this purpose.

Delusional parasitosis may be a shared illness in which some of the patient's close contacts also believe they too are infested. When two family members are involved, usually husband and wife or parent and child, the delusion is known as *folie à deux* ("a madness shared by two"). The psychological film *Bug* (2007) portrays a *folie à deux* involving a man and woman who believe they are infested with government-implanted, nano-technological insects.

Reassuring patients that no parasitic infestation exists can be difficult because they typically refuse to believe that their disease is functional rather than organic. Despite the outcome of laboratory tests that satisfy the doctor, patients frequently challenge and deny negative test results.

While management of drug-induced formication involves giving up the offending drug, referral for psychiatric therapy must be approached with tact and discretion.

Drugs that have been reported to cause formication include the following:

<u>Trade/Brand-names</u>

| Adderall | Ecstacy | Tridyl |
| Alcohol | Keppra | Wellbutrin |
| Cocaine | Lunesta | Zyban |
| Crystal meth | Ritalin | |

## Gustatory Hallucinations

A gustatory hallucination is a false or distorted perception of taste. The experience is often an unpleasant one, such as a persistent taste of metal.

# Chapter 4:
# Sleep Disorders

## Abnormal Dreams

> To sleep: perchance to dream: aye,
> there's the rub . . .
> —William Shakespeare,
>    *Hamlet,* Act 3, Scene 1

Dreams are a succession of images, ideas, emotions, and sensations that appear involuntarily to the mind during certain stages of sleep. Dreams, often a mixture of real and imaginary characters, places, and events, vary from the common and down-to-earth to the fantastic and surreal. I have described abnormal dreams as unusual, odd, bizarre, strange, or weird—unlike other "normal dreams" that the individual may have experienced in the past.

Sex dreams make up about 10 percent of all dreams, and sexual intercourse is the most common type of sexual content, followed by sexual proposals, kissing, and fantasies.

"Abnormal dreams" is an unofficial, fabricated, catch-all phrase used by the Food and Drug Administration (FDA) to describe one specific adverse side effect (out of more than 50,000 discrete adverse effects) of new generic drugs in medication trials. The *Medical Dictionary for Regulatory Activities* (MedDRA) is an international medical terminology system designed to support the classification, retrieval, presentation, and communication of medical information throughout the medical product regulatory cycle.

The medically adverse event classification dictionary is endorsed by and mandated in Europe and Japan for safety reporting. Its results are required to be listed in all Prescribing Information leaflets (Package Inserts) that pharmaceutical companies provide to physicians and, in a simpler, "dumbed-down" fashion, to pharmacists and patients. Although the term "abnormal dreams" has been expunged from medical literature since 2006, this side effect notation has, unfortunately, been perpetuated and still remains in virtually all Package Inserts past and present. The epithet "abnormal" has lost all its meaning . . .

The word *dream* is thought to have come from the Anglo-Saxon word meaning joy, gladness, or mirth. However, the word may have evolved from another word (from Sanskrit) meaning deception. When we dream, it is either a joy or a deception; Sigmund Freud was one of the first to emphasize dreams as keys to the unconscious. In his view, dreams are manifestations of repressed desires, usually sexual in nature.

Humans have always ascribed great significance to dreams, which have been variously viewed as windows to the hallowed, the past and the future, or the world of the dead. Sleep has often been induced by drugs or plants, whether opium, marijuana, peyote, kava kava, valerian, mescaline, or ketamine as well as dozens of other sleep-producing drugs or plants. These narcotics, which have the property of inducing rapid sleep and of heightening inward visions, make dreaming virtually instantaneous.

Dream interpretation was a prominent feature of the intellectual and imaginative world of late antiquity for martyrs and magicians, philosophers and theologians, polytheists and monotheists alike. The Sandman is a character in many children's stories, summoned to lull children to sleep. He sprinkles sand or dust on or into the eyes of the child at night to engender dreams and to ensure a restful sleep.


## Trivia:

- Blind people dream: People who become blind after birth can see images in their dreams. People who are born blind do not see any images, but have dreams equally vivid and often related to their other senses of sound, smell, and touch.
- Dreaming is not uniquely human. In 2001, in the journal *Neuron*, Massachusetts Institute of Technology researchers reported that cats, dogs, and other animals have complex dreams and are able to retain and recall long sequences of events while they are asleep.
- Ninety percent of dreams are forgotten within ten minutes of waking. Samuel Taylor Coleridge awoke one morning having had a fantastic dream after having taking some opium to which he had become addicted. He immediately began to compose his "vision in a dream" in what is one of English's most famous poems: "Kubla Khan." Partway through (at line 54) he was allegedly interrupted by "A person on business from Porlock." About an hour later, Coleridge returned to his poem but could not remember the rest of his dream. The poem was never completed.
- Alexander the Great, René Descartes, and Robert Louis Stevenson all claimed to have been directed by their dreams. Wolfgang Amadeus Mozart and Robert Schumann both declared to have first heard their compositions in their dreams. Johann Wolfgang von Goethe solved scientific quandaries and composed poetry in his dreams. The Israelites believed dreams to be messages from God.

- Giuseppe Tartini, the famous Italian violinist, composed his *Devil's Sonata* in 1713 under the influence of a dream. According to historical tracts, while fast asleep, Tartini dreamed that the Devil stood at the foot of his bed trying to bargain for his soul. So Tartini challenged the Devil to a musical duel. "How great was my astonishment," Tartini wrote, "when I heard him play with consummate skill a sonata of such exquisite beauty as surpassed the boldest flight of my imagination." When he awoke, Tartini, attempting to reproduce the netherworldly music of his dream, wrote *The Devil's Trill*, a sonata in G minor that is one of the finest pieces of music ever written; in short, a masterpiece.

- Every human being dreams, but men and women have different dreams and different physical reactions. Men tend to dream more about other men, while women tend to dream equally about men and women. In addition, both men and women experience sexually related physical reactions to their dreams regardless of whether the dream is sexual in nature; males experience erections and females experience increased vaginal blood flow.

- We only dream of what we know: Our dreams are frequently full of strangers who play out certain parts. They are real faces of real people that we have seen during our life but may not know or remember. The evil killer in your latest dream may be the man who sold you a bicycle when you were a child. We have all seen and spoken to thousands of faces throughout our lives; there is a limitless supply of characters for our brain to utilize during our dreams.

- Not everyone dreams in color. Twelve percent of sighted people dream exclusively in black and white; the remaining number dreams in full color. People also tend to have common themes in dreams. These themes include being chased, running slowly in place, sexual experiences, falling, arriving too late, someone dead now being alive, teeth falling out, flying, or failing an examination.

• People who have smoked cigarettes for a long time and then stop, have much more vivid dreams than they would normally experience. Dreams about smoking are the result of tobacco withdrawal, as 97 percent of subjects did not have them while smoking; their occurrence was notably related to the duration of abstinence. This type of a dream could be called wish fulfillment or a compensatory dream. The smoker misses smoking. He can not smoke during the day, and therefore he smokes in his dreams.

• When you are snoring, you are not dreaming.

• Toddlers do not dream about themselves until around the age of three. From the same age, children typically have many more nightmares than adults do until age seven or eight.

Chemicals in the brain, as well as life events, our own pre-occupations, and certain medications, influence our dreams. Medications reported to cause abnormal dreams include the following:

## Trade/Brand-names

| | | |
|---|---|---|
| Abilify | Chantix | Duragesic |
| Ambien | Cognex | Effexor |
| Aricept | Dalmane | Exelon |
| Avelox | Depakene | Epivir |
| Celexa | Depakote | Ketek |

## Trade/Brand-names

| | | |
|---|---|---|
| Lariam | Percocet | Sular |
| Lexapro | Permitil | Sustiva |
| Lipitor | Prevacid | Thorazine |
| Lopressor | Prialt | Toprol |
| Lortab | Prilosec | Toradol |
| Ludiomil | Prograf | Trizivir |
| Lunesta | Prolixin | Tussionex |
| Luvox | Prozac | Vfend |
| Malarone | Remeron | Viagra |
| Mellaril | Reminyl | Vicodin |
| Mirapex | Rythmol | Viread |
| Mobic | Sectral | Wellbutrin |
| Nicoderm | Serentil | Ziac |
| Nicorette | Seroquel | Zoloft |
| Nipent | Serzone | Zonegran |
| Norvasc | Singulair | Zyban |
| Norvir | Stelazine | Zyprexa |
| Paxil | Strattera | |

## Nightmares

> The waking have one world in common;
> sleepers have each a private world of
> their own . . . —Heraclitus

Nightmares are dreams that occur during rapid eye movement (REM) sleep, which cause a strong distressing emotional response from the sleeper, more often than not intense fear or horror, inescapable terror, extreme anxiety, agitation, or the sensations of pain, falling, drowning or death. Such dreams can be related to physical causes such as a high fever, or psychological ones such as anger, guilt, sadness, fear, anxiety, or depression. It frequently awakens the sleeper.

Nightmares are defined by four criteria:

- Sudden awakening from sleep with extreme fear and anxiety
- Immediate recall of the frightening content of the dream
- Full alertness on awakening with little confusion or disorientation
- Delayed return to sleep

The term *nightmare*, meaning a fearful awakening from sleep, appeared in the medical literature as early as 1753. In *An Essay on the Incubus or Nightmare*, John Bond describes nightmares as "seizing people sleeping on their backs, and often begin with frightful dreams that are soon succeeded by a difficult respiration, a violent oppression on the breast, and a total privation of voluntary movement . . . [after which] they are affected with strong palpitation, great anxiety, languor and uneasiness which gradually abate and are succeeded by the pleasing reflection of having escaped such imminent danger."

During the course of a nightmare, the sleeper may moan, talk, or move a little, although these signs do not always appear. The person awakens from the nightmare with a profound sense of fear. Waking is complete, and more often than not accompanied by increased heart rate, sweating, and other manifestations of anxiety or fear. Returning to sleep after a nightmare is often difficult. The intensity of the recall and the importance of the dream images in the person's mind can make it almost impossible to calm down and resume sleeping.

Many people experience nightmares when they are undergoing stress in their waking lives: difficulty on the job or with a loved one, moving, pregnancy, financial concerns, or after having suffered a traumatic event, such as surgery, the loss of a close relative, an assault, or a grave accident. Nightmares may also be triggered by major psychological traumas, such as those experienced by patients with post-traumatic stress disorder (PTSD). The nightmares of combat veterans fall into this category. The themes of these nightmares are typically

directly related to the traumatic event, and the nightmares often occur again and again.

Women have nightmares two to four times more frequently
than men. About 5 to 10 percent of adults have nightmares
once a month or more. Recurrent nightmares can interfere
with sleep and may cause people to seek medical help. Nightmares normally decrease in frequency as people grow older.

Causes of nightmares include the following:
- A major life event occurs before the nightmare in
  most cases
- Abrupt alcohol withdrawal
- Adverse reaction to or side effect of a drug (see list
  on page 70)
- Anxiety or stress (the most common cause)
- Breathing disorder in sleep (sleep apnea)
- Death of a loved one (bereavement)
- Eating just prior to going to bed; which raises the
  body's metabolism and brain activity
- Excessive alcohol consumption
- Illness with a fever
- Recent withdrawal from a drug, such as sleeping
  pills
- Sleep disorders (narcolepsy, sleep terror disorder)

The most frequent nightmare categories, in descending order,
were found to be as follows:
- Witnessing horror and violence
- Experiencing attack or danger
- Flight from someone or something
- A sinister presence
- Being late and frustrated in travel
- Suffocation
- Hallucinated creatures
- Being paralyzed

The most common theme is being chased. Adults are commonly pursued by an unknown male figure whereas children are usually stalked by an animal or some fantasy figure.

Nightmare was the original term for the state later known as *waking dream* (Mary Shelley and Frankenstein's *Genesis*), and more currently as sleep paralysis. Such nightmares were widely considered the work of demons and more specifically incubi, which were thought to sit on the chests of sleepers.

Folk belief in Newfoundland, South Carolina, and Georgia describe the negative figure of the Hag who leaves her physical body at night and sits on the chest of her victim.

In Charles Dickens' *A Christmas Carol*, Ebenezer Scrooge attributes the ghost he sees to "... an undigested bit of beef, a blot of mustard, a crumb of cheese, a fragment of an underdone potato. . ."

- Actress Winona Ryder has had a nightmare about children falling off a cliff and being unable to get to them in time.
- Madonna has said that she has a recurring nightmare that she's being attacked by a dwarf with a knife.
- Whitney Houston had recurring dreams of trying to cross the George Washington Bridge as it started to break apart.
- Horror-film legend Vincent Price was once asked to describe his worst nightmares. Price, an avid art collector, replied that they all involved his discovery that Leonardo DaVinci's *Mona Lisa* had been riddled with holes by someone's umbrella and left in a junk shop. "That," explained Price, "is really terrifying."

A nightmare can be a side effect of some medications or drugs of abuse, including drugs given for high blood pressure; levodopa and other drugs given to treat Parkinsonism, amphetamines, cocaine, other stimulants; and some antidepressants. Medications that have been reported to elicit nightmares include the following:

### Trade/Brand-names

| | | |
|---|---|---|
| Aldomet | Levatol | Sinemet |
| Aricept | Lipitor | Stadol |
| Axert | Ludiomil | Surmontil |
| Butisol | Marinol | Talwin |
| Capoten | Matulane | Tenormin |
| Catapres | Meberal | Thiopental |
| Chantix | Minipress | Timoptic |
| Cipro | MS Contin | Tofranil |
| Clozaril | Nicotine | Topamax |
| Codeine | Noctec | Toprol |
| Cymbalta | OxyContin | Vantin |
| Demerol | Pamelor | Vicodin |
| Dilaudid | Parlodel | Visken |
| Diovan | Paxil | Vitamin $B_3$ |
| Elavil | Pentobarbital | Vivactil |
| Ephedra | Phenergan | Wellbutrin |
| Fiorinal | Phenobarbital | Xanax |
| Imdur | Plaquenil | Zocor |
| Inderal | Proventil | Zoloft |
| Klonopin | Relafen | |
| Lanoxin | Serpasil | |

## Insomnia

> A flock of sheep that leisurely pass by,
> One after one, the sound of rain, and
>     bees murmuring;
> The fall of rivers, winds and seas,
> Smooth fields, white sheets of water, and
>     pure sky,
> I have thought of all by turns, and yet do lie
> Sleepless!
> —William Wordsworth

Insomnia, the difficulty in initiating or sustaining sleep, has been known for at least 2,000 years, as first recorded in Aristotle's thesis on sleeplessness in 350 BCE. Insomnia, the inability to get an adequate amount or quality of sleep, is a common symptom affecting millions of people. It is not a disease. It can be triggered by many conditions, diseases, or circumstances. At its most basic, insomnia can be defined as difficulty in falling asleep, staying asleep, or waking after too short a time.

Insomniacs, for a variety of reasons, find it very difficult to sleep. They feel they have no alternative but to quietly accept the fact that they will be fortunate if they are able to sleep even an hour or two at night. Insomnia is a nighttime sleeping problem. It may cause daytime problems, such as fatigue, lack of vitality, difficulty focusing, and irritability. Most adults have experienced insomnia at one time in their lives. An estimated 30 to 50 percent of the general population is affected by insomnia, and 10 percent have chronic insomnia. Insomnia can have a significant effect upon mood and hormonal activity and as a consequence can lead to depression, stress, and anxiety.

Meanwhile, all through the ages physicians have variously categorized insomnia as a symptom of deeper illnesses. In medieval and early modern times, physicians and philosophers held the theory that insomnia was a sign of lovesickness, sorrow, or even satanic possession. As modern medicine and science evolved, insomnia emerged as a distinct symptom of various disorders, such as post-traumatic stress disorder.

Symptoms associated with insomnia include the following:
- Co-existing medical and psychiatric illnesses
- Depression
- Difficulty with memory
- Headaches
- Heart disease (There is some evidence to suggest that severe insomnia can create activity within the heart and nervous system, which, in turn, could cause heart disease.)
- Impaired motor coordination

- Increased rate of accidents (Accidents at home, in the workplace and in particular on the road can often be traced back to insomnia sleep disorder.)
- Irritability and impaired social interaction
- Fatigue
- Poor concentration and focus
- Premature death (Strong evidence exists to show that individuals who frequently use sleeping pills have lower survival rates than the population as a whole.)
- Stress

Insomnia appears in several forms:
- Difficulty initiating sleep
- Early awakenings in the morning (before the desired time)
- Inadequate total sleep time
- Poor quality of sleep as reflected by its consequences, including daytime sleepiness
- Repeated or lengthy awakenings during the course of the night

Insomnia affects all age groups. Among older adults, insomnia affects women more often than men. The incidence increases with age. Insomnia may be a symptom of depression, and many people will have insomnia during the acute phases of a mental illness.

Certain groups are at higher risk for developing insomnia:
- Adolescent or young adult students
- People with chronic pain and cardiopulmonary disease
- Pregnant women
- Seniors
- Shift workers
- Travelers who experience jet lag
- Women in menopause

Sleep deprivation has often been used as a form of torture. In the Bible, God wished to test the character of Job. Part of his torment was severe insomnia: "When I lie down, I say, 'When shall I arise, and the night be gone?' and I am full of tossings to and fro unto the dawning of the day" (Job 7:4).

Throughout history, there have been many famous people who are known to have suffered from insomnia. In spite of the discomfort, frustration, stress, and tension and their inability to enjoy the benefits of a full night of deep, peaceful, relaxing sleep, these gifted individuals never permitted their insomnia to stand in the way of their dreams and plans—and they managed to achieve distinction in their chosen fields. Many of these famous people, compelled to cope with their sleep problems, also suffered from problems of depression and anxiety:

## Actors, Actresses, Singers:
- Cary Grant
- Marlene Dietrich: The only thing that lulled her to sleep was a sardine-and-onion sandwich on rye.
- Marilyn Monroe had been taking up to twenty phenobarbitals a day by the end of her life.

## Artists, Composers, Writers:
- Alexandre Dumas was one of the most creative insomniacs. He wrote enough words to fill 1,200 volumes and averred to have fathered 500 children.
- Charles Dickens—the position of his bed was an essential factor in reaching the sleeping state. He could only sleep in a bed that had its head pointing due north and then only if he lay precisely in the middle of the mattress.
- Evelyn Waugh used sleeping pills—although he was more often tormented by hallucinations instead of

achieving the suspended consciousness for which he longed.
- Marcel Proust was convinced that Veronal, a barbiturate, was the answer.
- Robert Burns, the Scottish poet, frequently referred to his inability to enjoy the comfort of a full night's sleep, and to his attacks of melancholy and anxiety.
- F. Scott Fitzgerald
- Shakespeare
- Vincent van Gogh could only fall asleep if he smothered his mattress and pillow with camphor so that he could clear his head of all his weird thoughts.
- Amy Lowell—whenever she stayed in a hotel, Lowell rented five rooms—one to sleep in, and empty rooms above, below, and on either side of her to ensure quiet.

## Historical Figures:
- Benjamin Franklin was more concerned with the temperature of his bed. He would get out of bed when unable to sleep and let it air and cool down. Then, when the sheets were cold, he would get back in to test it again.
- Margaret Thatcher had great difficulty in falling asleep.
- Napoleon managed to get by on as little as three hours of sleep.
- Sir Isaac Newton
- Thomas Edison had great difficulty in falling asleep and used to make up for his lack of nighttime slumber by dozing during the day.
- Winston Churchill suffered from insomnia for most of his life. He had twin beds, and when he couldn't fall asleep in one, he switched to the other one.

Certain medications have been associated with insomnia, among which are certain over-the-counter cold and asthma preparations. Medications for high blood pressure have also been associated with poor sleep. Common stimulants associated with insomnia include caffeine and nicotine. A list of those medications reported to cause insomnia include the following:

## Trade/Brand-names

| | | |
|---|---|---|
| Abilify | Aredia | Capoten |
| Accolate | Aricept | Carafate |
| Accupril | Arimidex | Cardene |
| Accutane | Arixtra | Cardizem |
| Aciphex | Aromasin | Cardura |
| Actifed | Asacol | Casodex |
| Actonel | Aspirin | Catapres |
| Adderall | Atacand | Ceclor |
| Adipex-P | Atrovent | Celebrex |
| Adrenaline | Avelox | Celexa |
| Adriamycin | Axert | CellCept |
| Aerobid | Axid | Celontin |
| Agrylin | Azactam | Cesamet |
| Aldara | Azulfidine | Chantix |
| Allegra | Bactrim | Chlor-Trimeton |
| Aloxi | Baraclude | Cialis |
| Alphagan | Benadryl | Cipro |
| Altace | Benicar | Clarinex |
| Ambien | Bentyl | Claritin |
| Aminophylline | Biaxin | Clinoril |
| Amitiza | Boniva | Clomid |
| Amoxapine | Bontril | Clozaril |
| Amoxil | Brethine | Codeine |
| Amytal | Butisol | Cognex |
| Anafranil | Calan | Colazal |
| Angiomax | Campath | Combipres |
| Ansaid | Campral | Compazine |
| Apokyn | Camptosar | Comvax |
| Aptivus | Cancidas | Cordarone |
| Arava | Cantil | Coreg |

## Trade/Brand-names

| | | |
|---|---|---|
| Corgard | Erbitux | Indocin |
| Cortisone | Estrogens | Inflenza vaccine |
| Cosopt | Ethmozine | Innohep |
| Cozaar | Eulexin | Intron |
| Crestor | Evista | Invanz |
| Cubicin | Evoxin | Invirase |
| Cymbalta | Exelon | Kerlone |
| Cytosar | Exjade | Ketek |
| Dacogen | Exovac | Klonopin |
| Dantrium | Extraneal | Kytril |
| Dapsone | Factive | Lamictal |
| Darvon | Fansidar | Lariam |
| Daypro | Faslodex | Lescol |
| Decadron | Felbatol | Leustatin |
| Deltasone | Feldene | Levaquin |
| Demadex | Femara | Levatol |
| Depakote+ | Flagyl | Levitra |
| Desoxyn | Flexeril | Levsinex |
| Didrex | Flomax | Lexapro |
| Dilantin | Floxin | Lipitor |
| Dilaudid | Flumadine | Lodine |
| Dimetane | Foscavir | Lomotil |
| Diovan | Frova | Lorabid |
| Dipentum | Fungizone | Lotensin |
| Ditropan | Fuzeon | Loxitane |
| Dolobid | Gabitril | Ludiomil |
| Dolophine | Gastrocrom | Lupron |
| Dostinex | Gemzar | Luvox |
| Duragesic | Geodon | Malarone |
| DynaCirc | Gleevec | Manurol |
| Effexor | Glucotrol | Matulane |
| Efudex | Gris-PEG | Mavik |
| Elavil | Haldol | Maxair |
| Eldepryl | Havrix | Meberal |
| Elmiron | HCTZ | Meclofenamate |
| Eloxatin | Herceptin | Medrol |
| Emcyt | Hyperstat | Meridia |
| Emtriva | Inderal | Meronem |

## Trade/Brand-names

| | | |
|---|---|---|
| Mevacor | OxyContin | Reyataz |
| Mexitil | Pamelor | Rhinocort |
| Miacalcin | Parlodel | Rilutek |
| Micardis | Parnate | Ritalin |
| Mifeprex | Paxil | Rituxan |
| Mirapex | PEG-Intron | Robaxin |
| Mobic | Pentobarbital | Robinul |
| Monopril | Pepcid | Rozerem |
| Motrin | Pepto-Bismol | Rynatuss |
| MS Contin | Permax | Rythmol |
| Mycobutin | Pertofrane | Sabril |
| Myleran | Phenergan | Salagen |
| Mylotarg | Plavix | Salgesic |
| Nalfon | Plendil | Sandostatin |
| Natrecor | Pletal | Seconal |
| Navane | Ponstel | Sectral |
| Nebilet | Pravachol | Serzone |
| Neoral | Prelone | Simulect |
| Neupro | Prevacid | Sinemet |
| Nexium | Prexige | Singulair |
| Nicotine | Prialt | Skelid |
| Nilandron | Prilosec | Soma |
| Nipent | Proamatine | Soriatane |
| Nolvadex | Procrit | Spectracef |
| Noroxin | Prograf | SPRYCEL |
| Norpace | Protonix | Stadol |
| Norvasc | Proventil | Strattera |
| Norvir | Provera | Stromectol |
| Novahistine | Provigil | Suboxone |
| Noxafil | Prozac | Sudafed |
| Numorphan | Rapamune | Surmontil |
| Nutropin | Reglan | Sutent |
| Nuvigil | Relafen | Symmetrel |
| Omnicef | Relpax | Synarel |
| Ontak | Reminyl | Synercid |
| Orap | Requip | Synthroid |
| Orudis | Rescula | Talwin |
| Oxsoralen | Revlimid | Tambocor |

## Trade/Brand-names

| | | |
|---|---|---|
| Tarceva | Tygacil | Wellbutrin |
| Targretin | Tykerb | Xeloda |
| Tavist | Tylenol | Xifaxan |
| Temodar | Tyzeka | Xopenex |
| Tenex | Ultram+ | Xyrem |
| Tenormin | Ultravist | Yohimbine |
| Tenuate | Valcyte | Zaditor |
| Teveten | Valium | Zantac |
| Thalidomd | Vantin | Zenapax |
| Thelin | Vaprisol | Zerit |
| Theo-Dur | Vascase | Zestril |
| Thyroid | Vasotec | Zevalin |
| Tikosyn | Velcade | Ziac |
| Tindamax | Ventavis | Zithromax |
| Tofranil | Viagra | Zocor |
| Tonocard | Vicodin | Zoladex |
| Topamax | Vidaza | Zoloft |
| Toprol | Vincasar | Zometa |
| Toradol | Viracept | Zomig |
| Torisel | Virazole | Zonegran |
| Tranxene | Viread | Zostavax |
| Trelstar | Visapaque | Zosyn |
| Trexan | Visken | Zovirax |
| Tricor | Vistide | Zyban |
| Trilafon | Vitamin $B_3$ | Zyflo |
| Trileptal | Vivactil | Zyprexa |
| Trisonex | Voltaren | Zyrtec |
| Trizivir | Vyvanse | Zyvox |

## Snoring

Snoring is the sound—soft, loud, and often disagreeable—of blocked air movement during breathing asleep. Snoring occurs when the flow of air through the mouth and nose is physically obstructed. The walls of the throat vibrate while breathing, resulting in the unique sounds of snoring.

At least 30 percent of adults snore. Snoring is known to cause sleep deprivation to both the snorer and those in earshot, as well as daytime sleepiness, lack of energy, poor motivation, high stress levels, irritability, lack of focus, decreased libido, and psychological and social harm.

Snoring may be genetic. Children who snore are almost three times as likely as others to have parents who snore. And snoring and sleep-disordered breathing are twice as common in children who test positive for allergies. Sleep-disordered breathing—snoring is one symptom of it—is linked to poor academic performance, cardiovascular troubles, and daytime behavioral problems such as attention-deficit hyperactivity disorder (ADHD). Elephants, pigs, dogs, cats, gorillas, and rhinos all snore.

Snoring taxes interpersonal relationships and causes embarrassment when snorers sleep outside their own homes. Snoring results in a poor night's sleep, which leads to drowsiness during the day and can interfere with the person's quality of life.

Spouses have lost untold hours of sleep from their partners' snoring. Vacations have been ruined and marriages destroyed by nighttime's most exasperating noise, a noise that can reach the decibel level of a diesel engine. The absolute threshold of human hearing is defined as 0 decibels (dB), and people with normal hearing can just begin to hear sound at 15 dB.

> Rustling leaves is about 10 dB.
> A whisper is about 20–30 dB.
> Normal conversation is about 60 dB.
> Most snoring registers in the range of 50–70dB.
> Busy street traffic is about 70 dB.
> Vacuum cleaners reach 80 dB.
> Chain saws and lawn mowers get to 90 dB.
> Large orchestra is 98 dB.
> Rock concert front row is 110 dB.
> Jackhammers hit 120 dB.

Threshold of pain is 130 dB.
A military jet takeoff attains about 140 dB.

Causes and associations with snoring:
- Alcohol and medications increase relaxation of throat and tongue muscles, making snoring more likely.
- Breathing problems such as asthma, upper respiratory, or sinus infections cause blockage in the nasal passageways and make inhalation difficult. This in turn creates a vacuum in the throat and noisy breathing.
- Being overweight can cause bulky throat tissue. Children with large tonsils and adenoids often snore.
- Deformities of the nose, such as a deviated septum (a structural change in the wall that separates one nostril from the other) or nasal polyps, can also cause obstruction and sleep problems.
- Fat accumulating in and around the throat can cause snoring.
- Heredity, such as inheriting a narrow throat, or any of the physical deformities mentioned above contributes to snoring.
- A long, soft palate or a long uvula (the dangling tissue in back of the mouth) can narrow the opening from the nose to the throat. When these structures vibrate and bump against each during sleep, the airway becomes obstructed causing snoring.
- Men have narrower air passages than do women and are more likely to snore.
- As people age, their throats become narrower and the muscle tone in the throat decreases.
- Misalignment of the jaw, often caused by tension in muscles, can contribute to snoring.
- Partially blocked nasal passages require extra effort to transfer air through them while sleeping. Some

people snore only during allergy seasons or when they have a sinus infection.

- Excess weight and fatty tissue in the neck cause the throat to become smaller.
- Throat and tongue muscles can be too relaxed, which allows them to collapse and fall back into the airway. Normal aging causes further relaxation of these muscles and increases the potential for snoring.
- Smoking or exposure to secondhand smoke relaxes muscles and also creates nasal and lung congestion.
- Throat weakness makes the throat close during sleep.
- Sleeping flat on the back allows the flesh of the throat to relax and block the airway.

Habitual snorers can be at risk for serious health problems:

- Lowered blood oxygen levels, causing the heart to pump harder and blood pressure to rise.
- Frequent waking from sleep, even though the person may not realize it.
- Long interruptions of breathing (more than ten seconds) during sleep caused by partial or total obstruction or blockage of the airway.
- Obstructive sleep apnea.
- Sleep Deprivation.

## Famous Snorers:
- Elizabeth Taylor
- Frank Gifford
- Howard Stern
- Michael Douglas
- Michelangelo
- Queen Victoria

- Regis Philbin
- Teddy Roosevelt (His snoring was so bad that when he once stayed in a Washington hospital, all the other patients had to be relocated to different floors so that they could sleep.)
- Winston Churchill

## Trivia:

Melvyn Switzer, a sixty-year-old British cabbie, is to snoring what Babe Ruth was to baseball, and is immortalized in the *Guinness Book of World Records:* On June 28, 1984, his snoring was measured at 87.5 decibels. Although Switzer is ranked as the champ, the British town crier Alan Myatt has been listed as the "World's Loudest Man" reaching an incredible snoring 112.8 decibels, about the same as a jet engine.

People have likened the scale and pitch of their partners' snores to a "pregnant rhinoceros," an "express train" and a "chain saw"; one particularly despondent participant described it as "hell as I imagine it to be."

About thirty million British adults are snorers. In the United Kingdom snorers are classified by the sound they make and Travelodge has compiled a list of the top five "snorer types":

1. The Snorter, distinguished by a rapid blowing of air through the nostrils and mouth, similar to the sound of a horse snorting
2. The Snorchestra, typified by long, low snores that gradually build into a deafening crescendo
3. The McEnroe, distinguished by violent grunting sounds, similar to the noise made by tennis stars when competing
4. The Walrus, typified by continuous groaning noises when sleeping

5. The Old Banger, sounds like a broken car
   with a spluttering engine
   Meanwhile, 20 percent of respondents who
   are in a relationship divulged that their snoring
   has had a negative effect on it.

In an extreme case of "snore rage," the notorious gunfighter, John Wesley Hardin, in 1871, is reported to have fatally shot a loud snorer in the next room.

A forty-three-year-old man has been accused of killing his hospital roommate after complaining that the man's snoring disturbed his sleep. In 1987, William Fitzmeyer was accused of either beating or strangling to death Thomas V. Fowler Jr., seventy-six, in the room they shared at Winthrop Community Hospital.

The study also found that as many as one in five children are guilty of nighttime rumblings and around one in three households have a pet that has a snoring problem.

Medications that have been reported to trigger snoring include the following:

### Trade/Brand-names

| | | |
|---|---|---|
| Catapres | Increlex | Xyrem |
| Diprivan | Sermorelin | |
| Fabrazyme | Versed | |

## Sleepwalking

### (Somnambulism; Noctambulism)

Sleepwalking (somnambulism) is a series of complex behaviors that are initiated during slow wave sleep (deep sleep or SWS) where the sufferer engages in activities that are, as a rule, associated with wakefulness while he or she is asleep or in a sleeplike state. About 20 percent of the population is prone to sleepwalking. While sleepwalking can affect people of any age, it is noted more in children than in adolescents and adults; boys are more likely to sleepwalk than girls are, and the highest prevalence of sleepwalking is at eleven to twelve years of age.

Sleepwalking is a sleep disorder; it is not a psychosis. It is more prevalent in people with high levels of stress, anxiety, or other psychological or genetic factors. Sleepwalkers are not conscious of their actions on a level where memory of the sleepwalking episode can be recalled, and because of this, unless the sleepwalker is wakened or aroused by someone else, this sleep disorder can be overlooked. Sleepwalking is not related to drug abuse but can be caused, albeit infrequently, by some medical conditions or by medications (see below).

Activities such as eating, bathing, urinating, dressing, driving cars, whistling, and committing murder have been claimed to have occurred during sleepwalking. Contrary to popular belief, most cases of sleepwalking do not consist of walking around; rather, they occur when the person is awakened, at which time the person may sit up, look around, and immediately go back to sleep.

The *Diagnostic and Statistical Manual of Mental Disorders* (DSM), a handbook for mental health professionals, specifies six diagnostic criteria for sleepwalking disorder:

- Significant breakdown of social and occupational situations, or other abilities to function.
- No impairment of mental activity upon waking.
- No recollection of the sleepwalking incident: (On waking, the person typically has no memory of the sleepwalking events.)
- Repeated episodes of rising from bed during sleep: Sitting up in bed, looking around, and walking.)
- Unresponsiveness to attempts at communication (The person has eyes open, dilated pupils, a blank stare, and does not respond to someone else's attempts at communication.)

Sleepwalking has in rare cases been used as a defense—occasionally successfully—against charges of murder. One successful incident occurred in Ontario, Canada, when Kenneth Parks was acquitted of all charges in 1987 for killing his in-laws, after evidence presented in his trial pointed to sleepwalking as the only possible explanation for his actions. However, in 1997, a Phoenix man who claimed to be sleepwalking when he savagely stabbed his wife 44 times to death was convicted of first-degree murder and was sentenced to life in prison.

Sleepwalking has been a theme in many dramatic works:

- It is a major plot element in the classic silent German Expressionist film *The Cabinet of Dr. Caligari* (1920). The title figure uses a haunting, zombie-like character—a somnambulist—as a circus attraction.
- Shakespeare's *Macbeth*. Lady Macbeth sleepwalks because of her overpowering guilt and insanity.
- Vincenzo Bellini's opera *La Sonnambula* is named after its heroine, a sleepwalker.
- In Dario Argento's *Phenomena* (1985), the protagonist, Jennifer Corvino (Jennifer Connelly), witnesses a murder while sleepwalking.
- In the film adaptation of *Silent Hill,* the protagonist's daughter suffers from sleepwalking.
- In the *House* episode "Role Model," a woman has sex with her ex-husband while sleepwalking and becomes pregnant.

Sleepwalking episodes can be very brief (a few seconds or minutes) or can last for thirty minutes or longer. Some people even drive a car while actually asleep. In a few instances, sleepwalking can result in savage behavior. While sleepwalking in children is not believed to be influenced by psychological factors, in adults, it could indicate a personality disturbance.

Sleepwalking episodes can range from sitting up in bed to walking, and can even lead to frantic attempts to escape as if threatened. During an episode, sleepwalkers may exhibit behaviors such as sitting up with glassy eyes, picking at the blankets, making body movements, and walking around the house. Sleepwalkers may also urinate, defecate, or avoid looking at another person who attempts to communicate or interact with them. Fleeing through a window is a familiar practice.

Symptoms of sleepwalking include the following:
- Sleeping with eyes wide open
- No memory of the episode when awakened
- Getting out of bed and walking around the room
- Mumbling incomprehensible phrases or talking nonsense
- Performing other acts—turning on the TV or cooking while asleep
- Sitting up while asleep
- Walking around with a blank expression
- When awakened, seeming confused and bewildered

Causes of sleepwalking:
- Alcohol consumption
- Drugs—prescription or recreational (see below)
- Fatigue
- Previous sleep loss
- Rapid Eye Movement (REM) disorders
- Worry and anxiety

Drugs that can give rise to somnambulism can include the following:

### Trade/Brand-names

| | | |
|---|---|---|
| Alcohol | Mellaril | Thorazine |
| Ambien | Noctec | Topamax |
| Depakote | Paxil | Trilafon |
| Halcion | Phenergan | Wellbutrin |
| Inderal | Restoril | Zyban |
| Lithobid | Sonata | Zyprexa |

# Chapter 5: Nervous System Disorders— Miscellaneous

## Convulsions

(Epilepsy; Seizures; Fits)

Since the beginning of time, it appears, epilepsy has affected millions of people, from beggars to kings. Epilepsy is one of the oldest conditions of the human race with a bountiful and distinguished history. The earliest references to epilepsy date back to the fifth millennium BCE in Mesopotamia, where epileptic auras, generalized convulsions, and other symptoms of what these ancient people called "the falling disease" were recorded with remarkably accurate descriptions. Ancient people thought epileptic seizures were caused by evil spirits or demons that had seized and invaded a person's body. Priests attempted to cure people with epilepsy by driving the demons out of them with magic and prayers. This superstition was challenged by ancient physicians like Hippocrates, who recognized a seizure as a dysfunction of the brain and not a paranormal or psychic event.

Today, epilepsy is known as a common, chronic neurological condition characterized by recurrent unprovoked epileptic seizures. It is also known as a *seizure disorder* and it is usually diagnosed after a person has had at least two seizures not caused by some known medical condition like alcohol withdrawal or extremely low blood sugar. Epilepsy is a common neurological disorder that can be diagnosed and treated with drugs and devices.

Epileptic seizures have a power and symbolism that, historically, have suggested an association with creativity or rare leadership skills. Scholars have long been intrigued by evidence that celebrated prophets and other holy men, political leaders, philosophers, and many who achieved prominence in the arts and sciences suffered from epilepsy.

One out of every hundred people in the United States has epilepsy. Their seizures arise from overly active neurons (nerve cells) in the brain. The rapid bursts of electrical signals emitted from these hyperactive neurons very briefly disrupt normal functioning, much like a lightning storm can interfere with electrical power in a neighborhood.

The hallmark of epilepsy is recurring seizures—sometimes as many as several hundred a day—under normal circumstances. In people with epilepsy, seizures can be triggered by something as trivial as lack of sleep or the flickering of a light.

What causes epilepsy in all cases is not known. In some people it results from the following:
- Brain damage incurred by a stroke
- Brain tumors
- Encephalitis
- Head injuries
- Lack of oxygen to the fetus during pregnancy, labor, or delivery
- Lead poisoning
- Measles
- Medications (see list on page 92)
- Meningitis

Epilepsy may run in families and can first appear at any age, although about 80 percent of all cases materialize during childhood.

There are more than twenty different types of epileptic seizures, ranging from the startling *grand mal* (also known as a serialized tonic-clonic) seizure to the slight few seconds loss of consciousness (known as an *absence* or *petit mal* seizure) that is often overlooked.

The emotional centers of the brain are often the most severely hit during a seizure, and a person suffering from epilepsy may start to cry for no apparent reason or become angry or afraid. These seizures are called *partial* because only part of the brain is involved. Many people misconstrue a person undergoing a partial seizure as drunk or suffering from a mental illness.

On the other hand, during a generalized seizure such as a *grand mal* seizure the whole brain is suddenly overloaded with added electrical energy so the entire body suffers convulsions and the person loses consciousness.

Some people experience a distinctive warning sign before a seizure, known as an *aura*. The aura is itself a form of partial seizure, but one in which the patient maintains awareness. It may be an odd smell, a cold breeze, a bright light, "butterflies" in the stomach, or hearing voices.

People who have suffered from epilepsy include:

## Actors, Actresses, Singers:
- Danny Glover: An actor and film director who had epilepsy from age fifteen to thirty-five.
- Bud Abbott: had epilepsy all his life, and tried to control and hide it by drinking.
- Ward Bond: was turned down from the draft in World War II.
- Margaux Hemingway: had epilepsy from the age of seven. Her death was attributed to suicide by an intentional overdose of phenobarbital, an anticonvulsant.
- Neil Young
- Richard Burton

## Artists, Writers, Composers:
- Vachel Lindsay
- Pyotr Ilich Tchaikovsky
- Lewis Carroll
- (Lord) George Gordon Byron
- Agatha Christie
- Hector Berlioz
- Leonardo DaVinci
- Edgar Allen Poe
- George Gershwin
- Georg Friedrich Handel
- Michelangelo
- Niccolò Paganini

## Sports Figures:
- Tony Lazzeri died after a probable seizure that occurred when he was alone at home.
- Florence Griffith Joyner developed seizures in her thirties and died from asphyxiation after a grand mal seizure while asleep.
- Grover Cleveland Alexander tried to hide his epilepsy with alcohol; at the time, alcoholism was considered to be a more socially acceptable problem than epilepsy.

## Notables with epilepsy have included:
- Alexander the Great
- Aristotle
- Fyodor Dostoyevsky
- Hannibal
- Napoleon
- Ida McKinley (First Lady of the United States from 1897 to 1901) had epilepsy in adulthood that became disabling and inconvenient. As was normal

for the time, great efforts were made to keep this secret.

- Ivan V Alekseyevich: (half brother of Russian Tsar Peter the Great) Ivan V was feebleminded, epileptic, and half-blind.
- James Madison
- Julius Caesar
- Martha Parke Custis, the daughter of Martha Washington and stepdaughter of George Washington, had seizures from early childhood and died during a seizure at age seventeen.
- Pope Pius IX had childhood epilepsy.
- Prince John: the youngest son of King George V, had epilepsy from the age of four until his death after a seizure at age thirteen. The shame of his epilepsy, along with other neurological problems, kept him from the public eye.
- Pythagoras
- Socrates
- Vladimir Lenin (first Premier of the Soviet Union) developed epilepsy late in life. His final year was characterized by neurological decline and loss of function. In his last few months, he developed epilepsy. His seizures worsened and he died in status epilepticus—a state of prolonged, generalized epileptic seizures in rapid succession with brief intervals of coma—which lasted fifty minutes.

Medications that have been reported to cause seizures include the following:

## Trade/Brand-names

Aciphex
Alfenta
Altace
Amerge
Amoxil
Azulfidine
Chlor-Trimeton
Codeine
Danocrine
Definity
Deltasone
DHT
Diamox
Dimetane

Diprivan
Elitek
Flumadine
Fungizone
Gastrocrom
Hepatitis vaccine
Imitrex
Inversine
Namenda
Neoral
Penicillin
Prelone
Provera
Reminyl

Serzone
Stadol
Tensilon
Tonocard
Topamax
Trileptal
Tylenol
Tylex
Ultram
Xylocaine
Zosyn
Zyrtec

## Depression

(BT) Depression—major depressive disorder—is a serious medical condition with a variety of symptoms. It is not just a short-lived mood, and it's not a sign of personal weakness. Symptoms can include sadness, feelings of guilt or worthlessness, restlessness, loss of interest in what was once enjoyed, and trouble concentrating or making decisions, as well as fatigue, vague aches and pains, headaches, and changes in weight or sleep patterns. Depression is often linked with a surge in the risk of suicide.

Depression is one of the leading causes of disability worldwide, and women are nearly twice as likely as men to experience it. People with a family history of depression may be more likely to develop this disorder. People with chronic medical conditions may also be vulnerable to the disease. A major life change can also increase the risk of succumbing to depression.

Depression affects about twenty million Americans in a given year or approximately one out of six adults over a lifetime. While many things may contribute to depression, its exact cause is not fully established. Certain chemicals called *neurotransmitters*—serotonin, norepinephrine, and dopamine—are thought to be involved in depression.

Medications that have been known to cause depression include the following:

## Trade/Brand-names

| | | |
|---|---|---|
| Accupril | Apresoline | Capoten |
| Accutane | Aralen | Cardene |
| Aceon | Arava | Cardizem |
| Aciphex | Aricept | Cardura |
| Actifed | Arimidex | Casodex |
| Actonel | Aromasin | Catapres |
| Adalat | Arranon | Celebrex |
| Adderall | Arsenic | CellCept |
| Adenocard | Asacol | Celontin |
| Adriamycin | Astelin | Cerebyx |
| Advair | Atacand | Cerubidine |
| Aerobid | Ativan | Cesamet |
| Agenerase | ATRA | Chantix |
| Agrylin | Avapro | Cipro |
| Aldara | Avelox | Claritin |
| Aldomet | Avonex | Clinoril |
| Aleve | Azilect | Clomid |
| Alfenta | Baclofen | Clozaril |
| Alphagan | Bactrim | Codeine |
| Altace | Beconase | Cognex |
| Ambien | Betapace | Coreg |
| Anafranil | Brevibloc | Corgard |
| Androgel | Brevital | Cosopt |
| Android | Butisol | Cozaar |
| Anectine | Calan | Crestor |
| Ansaid | Campath | Crixivan |
| Antivert | Campral | Crystapen |
| Apokyn | Cancidas | Cytosar |

## Trade/Brand-names

| | | |
|---|---|---|
| Cytotec | Faslodex | Lamictal |
| Dalmane | Felbatol | Lanoxin |
| Danocrine | Feldene | Lariam |
| Dantrium | Femara | Lescol |
| Darvon | Fiorinal | Levaquin |
| Daypro | Flagyl | Levatol |
| Decadron | Flexeril | Lexapro |
| Deltasone | Flomax | Lipitor |
| Demerol | Floxin | Lodine |
| Depakote | Fludara | Lomotil |
| Diamox | Flumadine | Loniten |
| Didrex | Forteo | Lopid |
| Didronel | Foscavir | Lotronex |
| Diovan | Frisium | Lozol |
| Dipentum | Frova | Lupron |
| Ditropan | Fungizone | Luvox |
| Dolobid | Fuzeon | Lyrica |
| Dolophine | Gabitril | Macrobid |
| Doral | Gastrocrom | Malarone |
| Dostinex | Gleevec | Marinol |
| Droperidol | Glucotrol | Matulane |
| Duragesic | Halcion | Maxair |
| DynaCirc | Haldol | Meberal |
| Effexor | HCTZ | Meclofenamate |
| Elavil | Herceptin | Meridia |
| Eldepryl | Hexalen | Meronem |
| Elmiron | Imitrex | Methazolamide |
| Elspar | Inderal | Mevacor |
| Emend | Intron A | Mexitil |
| Emtriva | Invanz | Miacalcin |
| Erbitux | Inversine | Micardis |
| Estrogen | Invirase | Minipress |
| Eulexin | Iopidine | Moban |
| Evista | Kenalog | Mobic |
| Exelon | Keppra | Monopril |
| Exovac | Kerlone | Motrin |
| Fansidar | Ketalar | MS Contin |
| Fareston | Klonopin | Myleran |

## Trade/Brand-names

| | | |
|---|---|---|
| Mylotarg | Plendil | Salagen |
| Nafcil | Ponstel | Sandostatin |
| Nalfon | Pravachol | Seconal |
| Nardil | Prevacid | Sectral |
| Nasonex | Prialt | Serpasil |
| Neoral | Prilosec | Simulect |
| Neurontin | Primaxin | Sinemet |
| Nexavar | Provigil | Singulair |
| Nexium | Progesterone | Soma |
| Nicotine | Prograf | Sonata |
| Nilandron | Proleukin | Spiriva |
| Nimotop | Prolixin | SPRYCEL |
| Nipent | Pronestyl | Stadol |
| Nizoral | Protonix | Suboxone |
| Nolvadex | Provera | Sudafed |
| Normozide | Quinora | Sufenta |
| Noroxin | Rapamune | Sular |
| Norpace | Reglan | Sustiva |
| Norvasc | Relafen | Sutent |
| Norvir | Relpax | Symmetrel |
| Novantrone | Remeron | Synarel |
| Nubain | Reminyl | Talwin |
| Numorphan | Requip | Tambocor |
| Nutrasweet | Revlimid | Tapazole |
| Nutropin | Rexitene | Tarceva |
| Nuvigil | Reyataz | Targretin |
| Orap | Rhinocort | Tasmar |
| Orudis | Rifamate | Tegopen |
| Oxsoralen | Rilutek | Tegretol |
| OxyContin | Risperdal | Temodar |
| Parlodel | Ritalin | Tenex |
| PEG-Intron | Rituxan | Tenormin |
| Pentobarbital | Robinul | Tensilon |
| Pepcid | Robitussin | Tenuate |
| Pepto-Bismol | Rozerem | Teveten |
| Periactin | Rynatuss | Thalidom |
| Phenergan | Rythmol | Tolectin |
| Plavix | Sabril | Tonocard |

## Trade/Brand-names

| | | |
|---|---|---|
| Topamax | Vascase | Xyrem |
| Toprol | Vasotec | Zanaflex |
| Toradol | Velban | Zanosar |
| Torisel | Vesicare | Zantac |
| Tranxene | Vfend | Zarontin |
| Travatan | Viagra | Zaroxolyn |
| Trecator-SC | Vicodin | Zelnorm |
| Trental | Vidaza | Zemplar |
| Trexa | Vincasar | Zenapax |
| Tricor | Viracept | Zetia |
| Trizivir | Virazole | Ziac |
| Trothane | Viread | Zocor |
| Tylenol | Visapaque | Zofran |
| Tysabri | Visken | Zoladex |
| Ultram | Voltaren | Zometa |
| Ultravist | Vyvanse | Zomig |
| Valcyte | Wellbutrin | Zonegran |
| Valium | Xanax | Zosyn |
| Valtrex | Xeloda | Zovirax |
| Vantas | Xylocaine | Zyrtec |

## Migraines

Migraine is a neurological disorder with a wide range of signs and symptoms. It is the most common neurological cause of a doctor's visit. Migraine headaches affect about thirty million Americans, and 75 percent of sufferers are women. Prepubertal migraine affects equal numbers of boys and girls. In addition to being a major cause of pain and suffering, chronic migraine attacks are a significant source of lost productivity and medical expenses.

About one-third of people who experience migraines get a preceding *aura*, in which a patient senses a curious light or offensive smell. Affecting about 20 percent of sufferers, and coming at the onset of an attack, these auras consist of flashing or shimmering lights, glittering sparkles, loss of vision, prickling and tingling over the face or arms, weakness, and speech problems.

Migraine usually leads to bouts of intense and debilitating headaches—often one-sided and pulsating—lasting anywhere from four hours to three days. They often occur with nausea and vomiting, a heightened sensitivity to bright lights, and noise. The word *migraine* is French in origin; it was Galen of Pergamum (129–216 CE), the most influential of all the physicians of antiquity, who used the term *hemicrania* (half head), from which the word *migraine* was derived.

Migraine is a disease; a headache is only a symptom. Migraine pain is caused by the expansion of the blood vessels in the brain; headache pain is caused by shrinking of the same blood vessels. During a migraine, inflammation of the tissue encircling the brain aggravates the pain. Medications often prescribed to treat a headache—such as beta-blockers—dilate the blood vessels and therefore can make a migraine worse.

Unlike most headaches, migraine has distinct stages, although not all sufferers experience each one. The phases of a migraine attack that are commonly experienced by many *migraineurs* (people who suffer from migraine) include the following:

- The *prodrome* occurs a few hours or days before the headache and consists of yawning, fatigue, sensitivity to light, and trouble in concentration.
- The *aura,* which immediately precedes the headache. This includes visual illusions and sparks of light.
- The *pain phase,* also known as the *headache phase.* Excruciating pain occurring with nausea, vomiting and sensitivity to light.
- The *postdrome,* which consists of lethargy, fatigue, difficulty focusing (the "zombie" phase), and persistent sensitivity to light.

Migraine attacks may be triggered by the following:

- Allergic reactions
- Bright flashing lights, loud noises, and certain odors, such as smoke or perfumes
- Physical or emotional stress
- Changes in sleep patterns
- Smoking or exposure to smoke
- Skipping meals
- Alcohol or caffeine
- Menstrual cycle fluctuations, birth control pills, and menopause
- Tension headaches
- Stress or time pressure
- Prolonged overexertion or uncomfortable posture
- Hunger or fasting

Common food triggers include the following:
- Aged cheeses
- Alcohol (red wine, Chianti, vermouth)
- Avocado
- Banana
- Caffeine products, as well as caffeine withdrawal
- Chicken livers
- Chocolate
- Citrus fruits
- Dairy products
- Fermented or pickled foods
- Figs
- Foods containing nitrates: bacon, hot dogs, and salami
- Foods with extremely high sugar content
- Monosodium glutamate (MSG)
- Nuts and peanut butter
- Onions
- Smoked fish

Headache with neuralgia was recorded in the medical documents of the ancient Egyptians as early as 1200 BCE. In 400 BCE Hippocrates described the visual aura that can herald the migraine headache and the relief that can take place through vomiting.

In the Middle Ages migraine was recognized as a distinct medical disorder with treatment ranging from hot irons to blood letting and witchcraft.

The conversion of Saul to Paul was a major event in the history of Western culture. The flashing light that caused Saul to fall down might be explained by a migraine. He had been suffering from one-sided headaches, as well as a chronic eye infection and photophobia (an abnormal sensitivity to or intolerance of light).

Famous migraine sufferers—*migraineurs*—past and present include the following:

## Actors, Actresses, Singers:
- Carly Simon
- Elizabeth Taylor
- Elle Macpherson
- Elvis Presley
- Loretta Lynn
- Star Jones
- Susan Olsen
- Frank Capra
- Fred Norris
- Howard Stern
- Jennifer Ringley
- Joan Didion
- Lee Grant

## Artists, Writers, Composers:
- Miguel de Cervantes

- Claude Monet
- Gustav Mahler
- Georges Seurat (after which is named the *Seurat effect*, a current medical term often used to describe the visual phenomena of scintillating aura)
- Vincent van Gogh
- Virginia Woolf
- Pyotr Ilich Tchaikovsky
- Lewis Carroll

## Sports Figures:
- Dwight Gooden
- Jose Canseco
- Kareem Abdul-Jabbar
- Se Ri Pak
- Scotty Pippen

## Historical Figures:
- Martin Luther King Jr.
- Mary Todd Lincoln
- Princess Margaret
- Robert E. Lee
- Napoleon Bonaparte
- Friedrich Nietzsche
- Blaise Pascal
- Charles Darwin
- Thomas Jefferson
- Ulysses S. Grant
- Joan of Arc
- Julius Caesar
- Karl Marx
- Sigmund Freud
- George Bernard Shaw

Medications that have been reported to trigger migraine headaches include the following:

## Trade/Brand-names

| | | |
|---|---|---|
| Abilify | Gabitril | Remeron |
| Aceon | Gastrocrom | Revlimid |
| Aciphex | Gleevec | Risperdal |
| Adriamycin | Havrix | Rituxan |
| Advair | IGIV | Sandimmune |
| Aerobid | Imitrex | Sandostatin |
| Agrylin | Intron A | Sonata |
| Anafranil | Lamictal | Soriatane |
| Arava | Levaquin | Sular |
| Asacol | Lexapro | Teveten |
| Botox | Lipitor | Thalidomid |
| Cardura | Miacalcin | Thelin |
| Celebrex | Micardis | Tikosyn |
| Chantix | Motilium | Topomax |
| Cialis | Neoral | Trileptal |
| Cipro | Neurontin | Tylenol |
| Claritin | Nexium | Ultram |
| Clomid | Nicoderm | Ultravist |
| Copaxone | Norvasc | Viagra |
| Coreg | Nuvigil | Viracept |
| Cozaar | Omniscan | Vitamin $B_3$ |
| Effexor | Orudis | Wellbutrin |
| Eldepryl | Paxil | Xopenex |
| Evista | PEG-Intron | Xyrem |
| Exelon | Percocet | Zelnorm |
| Exovac | Prevacid | Zoladex |
| Famvir | Protonix | Zyban |
| Felbatol | Proventil | Zyprexa |
| Flonase | Prozac | Zyrtec |

## Parkinsonism

Parkinsonism (also known as Parkinson's disease, shaking palsy, paralysis agitans, or PD), is a chronic and progressive degenerative disorder of the central nervous system that often compromises the sufferer's speech and motor skills.

Evidence suggests that Parkinsonism existed in ancient India and was described in the medical doctrine called *Ayurveda* as far back as 5000 BCE under the name *Kampavata*. The seeds of a tropical legume called *Mucuna Pruriens* (cowhage), containing about 4 percent levodopa, had been used in traditional Ayurvedic medicine to treat Parkinsonism centuries before this drug appeared in modern medicine.

The influential and prolific physician Galen, around 175 BCE, gave one of the first descriptions of this condition under the name *shaking palsy*. The malady, a result of the gradual destruction of cells in the brain responsible for producing and releasing the neurotransmitter—dopamine, was identified in 1817 by a physician, James Parkinson, who is credited with the first complete clinical description of the syndrome attributed to his name, Parkinson's disease. While most forms of Parkinsonism are of unknown origin, there are certain cases where the symptoms may result from toxicity, genetic alteration, head injury, other medical disorders, or medications (see list on page 104).

Parkinsonism is a disorder that affects nerve cells, or neurons, in the part of the brain that controls muscle action. In Parkinsonism, neurons that make dopamine die or do not operate properly. Dopamine normally sends signals that help to organize movements. Parkinsonism is characterized by muscle rigidity, tremor, a gradual slowing down of physical motility, and in extreme cases, a loss of physical movement. Other common symptoms include a shuffling gait with short steps, stooped posture, a masklike face with infrequent blinking, and fatigue. Depression is another common sign that occurs in 20 to 80 percent of cases.

Parkinsonism, a common *neurodegenerative disease* (a condition in which cells of the brain and spinal cord are lost) typically begins in the late fifties or sixties and occurs twice as often in men than in women. About one million people in the United States are afflicted with PD.

Famous victims, past and present, of Parkinsonism include the following:

## Actors, Actresses, Singers:
- Deborah Kerr
- Johnny Cash
- Jim Backus, he reportedly said of Parkinsonism, "you don't die from it, you die with it."
- Katherine Hepburn
- Michael Redgrave
- Terry-Thomas
- Vincent Price

One well-known sufferer of Parkinsonism is Michael J. Fox, who developed the disorder at age thirty. His book, *Lucky Man* (2000), focused on his experiences with the disease and his family's struggles in the midst of it. *Awakenings*, the film starring Robin Williams and Robert De Niro, is based on authentic cases reported by the popular author and neurologist Oliver Sacks.

## Artists, Writers, Composers:
- Salvador Dalí
- Eugene O'Neill

## Sports Figures:
- Muhammad Ali

## Historical Figures:
- Adolf Hitler

- Billy Graham
- Deng Xiaoping
- Eugene McCarthy
- Francisco Franco
- Douglas MacArthur
- Harry S. Truman
- Janet Reno
- Pierre Trudeau
- Pope John Paul II
- Yasser Arafat

Medications that have been reported to induce Parkinsonism include the following:

## Trade/Brand-names

| | | |
|---|---|---|
| Abilify | Geodon | Prolixin |
| Akineton | Haldol | Reglan |
| Amoxapine | Inapsin | Requip |
| Ancobon | Indocin | Risperdal |
| Azilect | Invega | Robitussin |
| BuSpar | Loxitane | Seroquel |
| Clopixol | Mellaril | Serpasil |
| Clozaril | Moban | Sinemet |
| Cogentin | Navane | Stelazine |
| Compazine | Neo-Synephrine | Symmetrel |
| Demerol | Orap | Thorazine |
| Depakene | Parlodel | Transderm-Scop |
| Depakote | Partane | Trilafon |
| Elavil | Paxil | Urised |
| Eldepryl | Permax | Urecholine |
| Exelon | Phenergan | Zyprexa |

## Restless Legs Syndrome (RLS)

Restless legs syndrome (RLS) is a common, chronic, neurological sleep disorder. The burning, creeping, and crawling sensations that are the hallmark of the disorder, lead to walking difficulties, sleep deprivation, and stress. It is a malady of the part of the nervous system that controls movements of the lower extremities and is characterized by the intractable urge to move the legs. It usually occurs or intensifies while resting; gets worse as the day wears on; and is often accompanied by pain or other troublesome sensations.

Often encountered in Parkinsonism, RLS affects about 8 to 10 percent of the U.S. population, and most people who are severely affected are middle-aged or older. This frequent disorder often goes unrecognized, is misdiagnosed and is poorly managed. In Germany alone eight million patients are affected by RLS, which makes it one of the most common neurological diseases. And in many people the condition is not diagnosed until ten to twenty years after symptoms begin.

While RLS, "the most common disorder you have never heard of," may have been known in antiquity, it has only lately come to medical attention. The earliest documentation of what was likely to be RLS occurred in 1685 and is credited to the well-known English physician, Thomas Willis, who served King Charles II. It was Willis who wrote "Instructions for Curing the Watching Evil," probably the first description of what we now know as RLS. In his publication, Willis writes, "the patients when being in bed exhibit leaping and contractions of the tendons and so great a restlessness and tossing of the members ensure, that the diseased are no more able to sleep, than if they were in the place of the greatest torture." In 1945, Professor Karl-Axel Ekbom identified, characterized, and coined the term "restless legs syndrome."

The International Restless Legs Syndrome Study Group has described the following symptoms of restless legs syndrome:

- Strange itching, "pins and needles," or "crawling" sensations occurring deep within the legs
- A compelling urge to move the limbs to relieve these sensations

- Involuntary, repetitive, periodic, jerking limb movements occur either in sleep or while awake at rest
- Restlessness—floor pacing, tossing and turning in bed, rubbing the legs
- Sleep disturbances and daytime sleepiness are very common
- Symptoms may occur only when lying or sitting

As minimal criteria for diagnosis, the group proposes the following four features:
- Desire to move the extremities
- Motor restlessness
- Worsening of symptoms at rest with some temporary relief by activity
- Worsening of symptoms in the evening or night

The severity of RLS symptoms ranges from mild to intolerable. Symptoms get gradually worse over time in about two-thirds of people with the condition and may be severe enough to be incapacitating.

RLS can be primary or secondary. Primary (idiopathic) RLS, far more common than secondary RLS, has no known underlying cause. In 25 to 75 percent of cases, primary RLS seems to run in families. Secondary RLS is caused by an underlying medical condition, such as the following:
- Pregnancy (About 40 percent of pregnant women experience RLS symptoms, which usually fade within a few weeks after delivery.)
- Chronic obstructive pulmonary disease (COPD)
- Chronic venous insufficiency or varicose veins
- Cigarette smoking
- Damage to the spinal nerves
- Fibromyalgia
- Hypothyroidism or hyperthyroidism
- Iron-deficiency anemia

- Lyme disease
- Parkinsonism
- Peripheral neuropathy, often a consequence of diabetes.
- Rheumatoid arthritis
- Stress and fatigue
- Uremia (kidney failure causing build up of toxins within the body.)
- Vitamin $B_{12}$ deficiency

Once the primary condition has been treated, secondary RLS will usually disappear without further medical care. It has been suggested that there is a strong relationship between RLS and major depressive disorder and/or panic disorder.

RLS is also known as "Jimmy Legs," under which name it was once featured in an episode of *Seinfeld*—Kramer's girl-friend suffered from it, and it was later revealed that George Costanza's mother was also a sufferer, although in actual fact, as George's father explained, she had "the Jimmy Arms . . . like you won't believe!" Another term often used for this disorder is "silly legs."

Medications or substances that can cause or aggravate RLS include the following:

## Trade/Brand-names

| | | |
|---|---|---|
| Alcohol | Intron | Sarafem |
| Caffeine | Iron | Seroquel |
| Celexa | Klonopin | Sinemet |
| Celontin | Lithobid | Topamax |
| Clozaril | Mirapex | Ultram |
| Dilantin | Neurontin | Xyrem |
| Dolophine | Paxil | Zoloft |
| Elavil | Prozac | Zonegran |
| Halcion | Remeron | Zyprexa |
| Haldol | Risperdal | |

## Paresthesia

### (Burning, Tingling, Prickling of the Skin)

Paresthesia is an abnormal sensation of tickling, tingling, prickling, or numbness of the skin with no obvious physical cause, more widely known as the feeling of "pins and needles." It occurs when an area of the body loses its normal sensation to touch. Transient paresthesia is usually caused by inadvertent pressure on a superficial nerve, which disappears slowly as the pressure is relieved. Other kinds of paresthesia, however, can be chronic and painful, and can result from a wide variety of sources. The feeling of having a foot "fall asleep" is a common one. This same combination of numbness and tingling can occur in any region of the body and may be brought about by a variety of disorders. Sensations such as these, which transpire without any associated stimulus, are called paresthesia. Other types of paresthesia include feelings of cold, warmth, burning, itching, and skin crawling.

Hands, fingers, and feet are common sites, but all areas of the body are vulnerable. In older people, paresthesia is often the result of poor circulation in the limbs.

Any type of tingling, burning, or numbness is usually a symptom related to a sensory nerve being damaged, diseased, or injured. Formication is a form of paresthesia. Causes depend on the exact location of the paresthesia sensations, but typically include a physical nerve injury or a disease condition affecting the nerves. If any of these tingling or numbness symptoms are more than just annoying, they can indicate a serious medical condition, such as multiple sclerosis, and call for prompt medical diagnosis.

Paresthesia can also be caused by and can be a symptom of the following conditions:
- Abscess
- Alcoholism
- Anxiety
- Arthritis

- Brain tumor
- Cancers
- Carbon monoxide toxicity
- Carpal tunnel syndrome
- Circulatory disorders
- Dehydration
- Diabetes
- Fibromyalgia
- Herniated disc
- Herpes zoster (shingles)
- Hyperventilation
- Hypoparathyroidism
- Lead poisoning
- Leprosy
- Low blood sugar (hypoglycemia)
- Lupus
- Malnutrition
- Mental stress
- Migraines
- Multiple sclerosis
- Nerve compression
- Nerve injury
- Neuropathy
- Panic attacks
- Peripheral neuropathy
- Pernicious anemia
- Pinched nerve
- Rheumatoid arthritis
- Sleeping on a nerve
- Spinal cord disorders
- Thyroid problems
- Tobacco use
- Transient ischemic attack (commonly called a mini-stroke)
- Tumors
- Vitamin $B_{12}$ deficiency

- Vitamin $B_5$ deficiency
- Whiplash injury
- Withdrawal from certain selective serotonin reuptake inhibitors (SSRI antidepressants), such as Celexa, Lexapro, Prozac, Luvox, Paxil, Zoloft, etc.

Drugs that are commonly associated with paresthesias include the following:

## Trade/Brand-names

| | | |
|---|---|---|
| Accupril | Aromasin | CellCept |
| Accutane | Arranon | Cerebyx |
| Aceon | Arsenic | Cesamet |
| Aciphex | Asacol | Chemet |
| Actifed | Astelin | Cialis |
| Adenocard | Atacand | Cipro |
| Adriamycin | Atarax | Claritin |
| Advair | Atrovent | Clinoril |
| Agenerase | Avapro | Cocaine |
| Aggrenox | Avelox | Comvax |
| Agrylin | Axert | Concerta |
| Aleve | Azactam | Coreg |
| Aloxi | Azilect | Cosopt |
| Altace | Baclofen | Coumadin |
| Ambien | Benadryl | Cozaar |
| Amerge | Betapace | Crestor |
| Amitiza | Brevibloc | Crixivan |
| Amoxapine | BuSpar | Cubicin |
| Anafranil | Calan | Cymbalta |
| Ancobon | Campral | Cytovene |
| Androgel | Camptosar | Danocrine |
| Ansaid | Capoten | Daypro |
| Antivert | Cardene | Desferal |
| Anzamet | Cardizem | Depakene |
| Arava | Cardura | Depakote |
| Aredia | Casodex | Diamox |
| Aricept | Ceclor | Didronel |
| Arimidex | Celebrex | Dilantin |

## Trade/Brand-names

| | | |
|---|---|---|
| Dimetane | Hycamtin | Miacalcin |
| Diovan | Hygroton | Micardis |
| Dipentum | Hyzaar | Migranal |
| Diprivan | Imitrex | Miltown |
| Diuril | Inderal | Minipress |
| Dolobid | Indocin | Minocin |
| Dopram | Insulin | Mitomycin |
| Dostinex | Intron A | Mobic |
| Duragesic | Invanz | Monopril |
| DynaCirc | Invirase | Monurol |
| Effexor | Iopidine | Namenda |
| Elavil | Keppra | Natrecor |
| Eldepryl | Kerlone | Nebilet |
| Elitek | Ketek | Neoral |
| Enbrel | Lamictal | Neupro |
| Exelon | Lariam | Neurontin |
| Exovac | Lasix | Nexium |
| Factive | Lescol | Niacinamide |
| Famvir | Levaquin | Nicotine |
| Faslodex | Levitra | Nipent |
| Felbatol | Lexapro | Nizoral |
| Femara | Lipitor | Nolvadex |
| Fiorinal | Lodine | Normozide |
| Flexeril | Lopid | Noroxin |
| Fludara | Lotensin | Norpace |
| Foscavir | Lunesta | Norvasc |
| Frova | Lupron | Norvir |
| Fungizone | Luvox | Novahistine |
| Gabitril | Lyrica | Nuvigil |
| Gastrocrom | Macrobid | Ofloxin |
| Gemzar | Marplan | OxyContin |
| Geodon | Matulane | Pamelor |
| Gleevec | Mavik | Panretin |
| Glucotrol | Meridia | Parlodel |
| Gris-PEG | Meronem | Parnate |
| Halcion | Methazolamide | Paxil |
| Herceptin | Mevacor | Pepcid |
| Humira | Mexitil | Periactin |

## Trade/Brand-names

| | | |
|---|---|---|
| Pertofrane | Sinemet | Toradol |
| Plavix | Sinequan · | Tricor |
| Plendil | Singulair | Trizivir |
| Pravachol | Skelid | Trusopt |
| Prevacid | Somavert | Tylenol |
| Prezista | Sonata | Ultracet |
| Prialt | Soriatane | Ultram |
| Prilosec | Spiriva | Ultravist |
| Primaxin | Stadol | Valcyte |
| Proamatine | Streptomycin | Vascase |
| Procrit | Suboxone | Vasotec |
| Progesterone | Sular | Velban |
| Prograf | Sumycin | Velcade |
| Propylthiouracil | Surmontil | Vfend |
| ProSom | Sustiva | Viagra |
| Protonix | Symmetrel | Vicodin |
| Provera | Synarel | Vincasar |
| Provigil | Synercid | Viracept |
| Ranexa | Talwin | Viramune |
| Rapamune | Tambocor | Visipaque |
| Regitine | Tapazole | Visken |
| Relafen | Tarceva | Vistaril |
| Relpax | Targretin | Vitamin $B_{12}$ |
| Remeron | Tarka | Vitamin $B_3$ |
| Reminyl | Tasmar | Vitamin $B_6$ |
| Remodulin | Temodar | Voltaren |
| Requip | Teslac | Wellbutrin |
| Revlimid | Testosterone | Xanax |
| Rhinocort | Tetracycline | Xeloda |
| Ritalin | Teveten | Xoponex |
| Rituxan | Thalidomid | Xylocaine |
| Romazicon | Tikosyn | Zanaflex |
| Rythmol | Timoptic | Zaroxolyn |
| Sabril | Tobrex | Zavesca |
| Salagen | Tofranil | Zestril |
| Sandostatin | Tonocard | Zetia |
| Serzone | Topamax | Ziac |
| Simulect | Toprol | Zithromax |

## Trade/Brand-names

| | | |
|---|---|---|
| Zocor | Zomig | Zyloprim |
| Zofran | Zonegran | Zyprexa |
| Zoladex | Zostavax | Zyrtec |
| Zoloft | Zovirax | |
| Zometa | Zyban | |

## Suicidal Ideation

> There is but one truly serious question,
> and that is suicide.
> — Albert Camus, *The Myth of Sisyphus*

Suicidal ideation includes all thoughts of suicide, both when the thoughts include a plan to commit suicide and when they do not include a plan; it is one of the symptoms of both major depression and bipolar depression. Suicidal ideation is more common than completed suicide. Most persons who commit suicide have a psychiatric disorder at the time of death. The majority of patients with suicidal ideation do not in the end commit suicide. Attempted suicides, resulting in injury, hospitalization, and/or emotional and mental trauma, amount to ten to twenty times the number of successful suicides.

The overall suicide rate is 11 per 100,000 persons, ranking suicide as the ninth leading cause of death. In the United States alone, someone dies by suicide once every seventeen minutes and suicide is the third leading cause of death for youths between the ages of fifteen and twenty-four. Every thirty seconds someone in the world commits suicide.

Suicide is responsible for almost half of all violent deaths, amounting to almost one million fatalities every year. Worldwide, more people die from suicide than from all homicides and wars combined. In most European countries, the number of suicides each year is greater than the number of traffic deaths. Among reporting countries, the highest rates of suicide are in

Eastern Europe, while the lowest rates are in Latin America, Muslim countries, and a few Asian countries.

Causes of suicidal behavior include the following:

• Arguments
• Breakdowns in relationships
• Legal or work-related problems
• Loss of loved ones
• Poverty
• Unemployment

A family history of suicide, as well as alcohol and drug abuse, childhood abuse, social isolation, and some mental disorders, including depression and schizophrenia, also play a central role in a large number of suicides. Physical illness and disabling pain increases suicide risks.

There is no "typical suicidal person." However, the following behaviors may suggest that a person is seriously considering suicide.

• Drastic change in behavior and taking unnecessary risks
• Increased use of alcohol and drugs
• Loss of interest in work, school, or hobbies and withdrawal from social activities, friends, and family
• Signs of preparing for death such as making funeral arrangements or giving away prized possessions
• Talk about committing suicide and preoccupation with death and dying
• Trouble eating or sleeping and noticeable change in personal appearance

Although 80 percent of persons who commit suicide are men, the majority of those who make nonfatal suicide attempts are women between twenty-five and forty-four years of age. A previous suicide attempt is considered the best predictor of a completed suicide.

In urban legends, suicide attempts *always* have an ironic outcome—as in the familiar (but untrue) tale of the man who was dismissed from his job and jumped from his office window intending to kill himself, only to land on and kill his former employer on the sidewalk below.

## Celebrity Suicides:

- Hart Crane, poet 1932—suicide by drowning. On a steamship, he bid his fellow passengers farewell and jumped overboard.
- Joseph Goebbels, Nazi politician 1945—with his wife, he poisoned their five children, then committed suicide at Hitler's Berlin bunker.
- Jim Jones, leader of a religious cult known as the Peoples Temple 1978—killed himself after watching more than 900 of his followers die from the ingestion of Kool-Aid laced with cyanide.
- Nero, Roman emperor 68 BCE—committed suicide by stabbing himself with a sword.
- Sylvia Plath, poet, committed suicide by inhaling gas from her oven.
- Socrates, philosopher 399 BCE—was ordered to drink hemlock to end his life after being found guilty of corrupting the youth of Athens.
- Vincent van Gogh, artist 1890—shot himself; he died two days later.
- Virginia Woolf, writer 1941—committed suicide by drowning.

In a 2008 study, the FDA showed that patients receiving antiepilepitic drugs had amost twice the risk of suicidal behavior or ideation compared to those patients receiving placebos. The drugs included in the analyses included Tegretol, Felbatol, Neurontin, Lamictal, Keppra, Trileptal, Lyrica, Gabitril, and Topamax.

Medications that can cause suicide ideation include the following:

## Trade/Brand-names

| | | |
|---|---|---|
| Abilify | Isordil | Sandostatin |
| Ambien | Keppra | Sarafem |
| Amoxapine | Lamictal | Serax |
| Anafranil | Lariam | Seromycin |
| Anthrax vaccine | Lexapro | Seroquel |
| Avelox | Librium | Serzone |
| Aventyl | Ludiomil | Sinequan |
| Avonex | Luvox | Sonata |
| Azilect | Lyrica | Strattera |
| Campral | Marijuana | Sustiva |
| Celexa | Marplan | Symmetrel |
| Celontin | Meridia | Tegretol |
| Chantix | Mysoline | Tequin |
| Clomid | Namenda | Thlidomid |
| Cocaine | Nardil | Tofranil |
| Cymbalta | Neurontin | Topamax |
| Decadron | Nizoral | Trileptal |
| Depakene | Pamelor | Ultracet |
| Depakote | Parnate | Ultram |
| Desyrel | Paxil | Vaniqa |
| Diamox | Peganone | Viracept |
| Dilantin | Pertofrane | Vivactil |
| Ecstacy | Phenobarbital | Vivitrex |
| Effexor | Prialt | Wellbutrin |
| Elavil | Proleukin | Xyrem |
| Eldepryl | Prozac | Zagam |
| Ephedra | Q-Vel | Zanaflex |
| Eskalith | Rebetron | Zarontin |
| Felbatol | Reglan | Zelnorm |
| Fuzeon | Remeron | Zoloft |
| Gabitril | Remicade | Zonegran |
| Geodon | Reminyl | Zyban |
| Imdur | Requip | Zyprexa |
| Intron | Risperdal | Zyrtec |
| Invirase | Sabril | |

# PART B
# SKIN AND HAIR
# DISORDERS

## Chapter 1: Skin

### Acne

> "There is no single disease which causes
> more psychic trauma, more maladjust-
> ments between parents and children,
> more general insecurity and feelings of
> inferiority and greater sums of psychic
> suffering than does acne."
> — Sulzberger & Zaldems, 1948

Acne, the scourge of adolescence, is more than skin deep.
There are few skin ailments that cause as much physical and
psychological anguish as this complex chemical mystery that
affects almost twenty million people in the United States. The
market for prescription and over-the-counter acne medications

is well over $1.5 billion a year. And there are no quick, magical cures for it.

By far the most common teenage skin disorder, acne usually begins at puberty, a time when oil glands in the skin enlarge and increase the production of skin oil (sebum). This occurs as a result of rising hormones during adolescence. Ranging from simple pimples to angry boils, these unsightly blemishes will plague nine out of ten pubertal youngsters at an age when physical attractiveness becomes so important.

Acne appears most frequently in the mid-teens when hormone levels increase and kick the skin's oil gland into overdrive, but they can become present as early as the ninth year. It usually continues into the twenties. It may appear transiently in the newborn and is often seen in women in their midthirties. The incidence of acne in adult women is now more than 50 percent, compared to 35 percent in 1979.

The condition appears earlier in girls but is more frequent and more severe in boys. Overall, Blacks and Asians tend to have fewer and less severe acne problems. Acne can be hereditary; parents who had severe acne during their teenage years often have children who develop severe acne.

Acne occurs on areas of the body where oil glands are the largest, most numerous and most active: the face, chest, and back. Simply stated, these enlarged and overactive oil glands become clogged with oil and sticky skin cells, thus forming blackheads and whiteheads. (When a skin pore is closed and oil can't escape, the swelling is called a whitehead; when the skin pore isn't closed but is simply plugged up with dead cells and oil, it's called a blackhead. The dark color of the blackhead is *not* due to dirt: it is a result of pigment cells—melanin—in the upper layers of the skin.)

The glands continue to manufacture oil that is unable to escape. Bacteria, which are always on the skin in "friendly" and harmless numbers, set up housekeeping and begin to thrive in these trapped secretions. They then become "unfriendly" and harmful, causing infected pimples, or "zits." These zits may lead to cysts (little sacs filled with fluid or cheesy material), which then break down to form scars.

Other factors that can aggravate acne include hormonal disorders as well as medications such as cortisone, iodides, lithium, and anti-epilepsy medications (see below). Young men who are taking anabolic steroids for bodybuilding are prone to the severe cystic type of acne that doesn't respond to conventional anti-acne medications. Young women often experience acne eruptions just before their menstrual periods. The "low-dose" birth control pills also are responsible for acne in women who never had the problem as adolescents. Many women note a worsening—even an onset—of acne two or three months after having discontinued their oral contraceptive. This phenomenon can last as long as two years. Excessive brushing with a hairbrush or hair dryer attachment may cause persistent localized acne over the temple and forehead. Nuts and peanut butter, as well as excesses of dairy products, have been reported by many dermatologists recently as initiating and aggravating acne breakouts.

Several noted celebrities have had acne:
- Alicia Silverstone
- Angelina Jolie
- Billie Piper
- Brad Pitt
- Britney Spears
- Cameron Diaz
- Jessica Simpson
- Leonardo DiCaprio

A few notes on zits:
- A "zit" is a common, colloquial expression that young people often use when referring to an acne "bump" or pimple. These "bumps," or zits, come in many sizes, and, depending upon how large they are, can go by a variety of other names. The common, everyday, garden-variety is about the size of a pea.

- A larger zit—the size of a small grape—is called a "goober." So if you have lots of "zits and goobers," you usually have a face full of acne: a "pizza face."
- When the "goober" becomes very large—say, the size of a large cherry—I call it a "zinger." And then there's the "honker." This is the "third eye" you wake up with the morning of the prom.
- Finally, we have the "screamer." This is when your mother sees you first thing in the morning with a monstrous, walnut-sized lump on your cheek and lets out a tremendous scream!
- Then, of course, there are the "splashers," but I won't elaborate on these; you can probably guess what they are.

## Acne—Common Myths & Misconceptions:

Myth #1: Acne is a disease of adolescence. While it is true that acne usually appears during puberty, this is not always the case. Many people, particularly women, don't develop acne until their twenties or thirties, and it can afflict both men and women well into their forties.

Myth #2: Acne is more common in girls. Young women are more likely to see a dermatologist about their acne problems because they are generally more conscious of their appearance. However, acne affects both sexes. In fact, the severe cystic form of acne of the back is more common in men.

Myth #3: Acne is due to improper hygiene.

In reality, acne patients generally are more fastidious and conscientious about cleanliness than other teenagers. Blackheads, the primary hallmark of acne, do not result from dirt but from pigment (melanin) in the oil glands.

Myth #4: Masturbation causes or aggravates acne.
The only link between masturbation and acne is that both are often associated with adolescence. Moralists of the nineteenth century blamed many diseases on such "sinful" practices. The guilt surrounding masturbation in the minds of many teenagers probably perpetuates this timeworn myth.

Myth #5: Sexual intercourse will cure acne.
While this form of therapy sounds appealing, there is no evidence to document that it works. This belief probably stems from an old European myth that marriage cures acne. People often got married in their early twenties— about the same time that acne usually burns itself out.

Medications that have been known to cause and/or aggravate acne include the following:

### Trade/Brand-names

| | | |
|---|---|---|
| Adriamycin | Android-F | Celestone |
| Aerobid | Antabuse | CellCept |
| Amoxapine | Arava | Cerebyx |
| Anafranil | Asacol | Cipro |
| Andro | Brevibloc | Clomid |
| Androgel | BuSpar | Cognex |
| Android | Carteol | Cortone |

## Trade/Brand-names

| | | |
|---|---|---|
| Cosmegen | Mesantoin | Relafen |
| Cymbalta | Myleran | Remeron |
| Cytovene | Nalfon | Rheumatrex |
| Danocrine | Neoral | Risperdal |
| Dantrium | Nexavar | Sandostatin |
| Deltasone | Nexium | Serzone |
| Dilantin | Nicotrol | Simulect |
| Dostinex | Nimotop | SPRYCEL |
| Eldepryl | Nipent | Sular |
| Emend | Parnate | Synarel |
| Erbitux | Paxil | Tapazole |
| Felbatol | Pepcid | Targretin |
| Flonase | Pertofrane | Tegretol |
| Gold | Prelone | Thalidomid |
| Haldol | Premarin | Topamax |
| Herceptin | Prevacid | Trecator |
| Heroin | Priftin | Trexan |
| Inderal | Progesterone | Tricor |
| INH | Prograf | Trileptal |
| Inverase | ProSom | Tysabri |
| Iressa | Protonix | Valium |
| Kenalog | Provera | Vaniqa |
| Kerlone | Prozac | Vectibix |
| Lamictal | Pulmicort | Vistide |
| Lipitor | Pyrazinamide | Xyrem |
| Loniten | Quinine | Zanapax |
| Lupron | Quinora | Ziac |
| Luvox | Rapamune | Zonegran |
| Medrol | Raptiva | Zyrtec |

## Hives

(Urticaria)

> A disorder of hidden cause and unpre-
> dictable course. — Jerome Z. Litt

Hives is a very common disorder and has been known as a disease since antiquity. At least 20 percent of the general population will develop some form of hivelike eruption in the course of a lifetime. Fortunately, most episodes last for a few days to a couple of weeks and the cause, in these cases, is often promptly identified.

Contrary to popular opinion, hives is *not* a disease. Caused by the release of a chemical called histamine, hives—*urticaria*—is a symptom of some disorder or allergic mechanism in the body. Hives pop up on the skin and mucous membranes in the form of itching, stinging, and burning wheals (welts), surrounded by an area of redness. They look like big mosquito bites. New patches develop as old ones fade away. Hives come in a variety of sizes and shapes and can appear just about anywhere on the body, but mostly on pressure points where one sits or leans.

When the wheals are very large and the loose tissue of the eyelids, lips, and tongue swell up, the condition is called *angioedema*, or *bull hives*. Hives may involve the mucous membranes of mouth and throat, and in rare cases may even obstruct breathing so severely that heroic medical methods are necessary to prevent suffocation.

Like coughing or sneezing, which may signal a response to an upper respiratory infection or hay fever, hives are a clue, alerting us to abnormal goings-on in our system. For example, hives may be a response to an infection, an allergic reaction to some strange food or drug, or the result of emotional tension. It is extremely difficult to pinpoint the specific cause of a case of hives, mainly because the possibilities are endless. In the acute type of hives—where the itching and wheals appear quickly and fade in a few minutes or hours—it is somewhat easier to uncover the culprit: a strange food, an emotional upset, a penicillin injection, a new medication, or some recent infection such as chicken pox, mononucleosis, or an upper respiratory ailment.

Unfortunately, in the chronic form—which occurs most commonly in middle-aged women, and which may last for months or even years—the culprit is much more difficult to determine.

The most common causes of hives are certain foods and drugs. Strawberries, nuts, chocolate, fish and shellfish, milk, eggs, pork, oranges, bananas, and many other edibles, such as the artificial sweeteners saccharin and aspartame, can cause hives. Hives can appear within minutes or up to two hours after eating an allergenic food.

Some people get hives from inhaling substances such as animal dander (from cats, dogs, or horses), house dust, pollen, molds, certain plants, or flour. Others break out in hives when they touch something cold or something hot, and still others when they are exposed to sunlight. Some even get hives when pressure is applied to their skin, as in the shower.

There are certain types of hives that are of psychogenic origin in response to fear, anger, and stress.

Underlying infections of the teeth, sinuses, gastrointestinal, respiratory, and genitourinary tracts all can cause hives. Hives are also associated with untreated athlete's foot and viral diseases such as hepatitis and infectious mononucleosis.

Finding the cause of chronic, recurrent hives is often a difficult, frustrating, and lengthy process, and requires patience and extensive detective work. Only when you are able to discover the cause, can you prevent your hives from recurring.

- The earliest description of the disease we today call urticaria is found in *The Yellow Emperor's Inner Classic*, which was probably written in the first century BCE. In Chinese, urticaria is called *Feng Yin Zheng,* which means "wind-type concealed rash."
- Hippocrates (460–377 BCE) described elevated itching lesions caused by nettles, which he called *knidosis* after the Greek word for nettle (*knido*).
- Thomas More, in his book *King Richard III,* gives an excellent description of the condition without giving it a name presenting the first recorded case

of urticaria reported to cause death. In 1480 before his coronation, King Richard surreptitiously ate some strawberries just prior to giving an audience to Lord William Hastings and promptly developed acute urticaria. Assembling the lords, he opened his shirt and showed his chest, which was covered with red elevated and itching spots. He then accused Hastings of putting a curse on him and had him assassinated on the spot.

Although the word *urticaria* was first introduced in 1769, nettle rash was still in vogue until the early 1960s.

Medications that commonly cause hives include antibiotics, sedatives, tranquilizers, vitamins, laxatives, and dozens more. Of the various drugs and medications, penicillin is probably the most common cause. If you are allergic to penicillin and suffer from hives, you should avoid milk and certain cheeses, such as blue cheese and Roquefort. Milk and other dairy products may contain enough penicillin to prolong hives for years. The systematic use of other antibiotics, such as tetracycline, in cattle feed also can cause hives.

Sulfa drugs (sulfonamides) are notorious for causing hives. If you are allergic to sulfa (not sulfur), you should know that many common compounds contain sulfa. Saccharin and the "thiazide" diuretics—Lasix, Dyazide, hydrochlorothiazide, Prinizide, and others—as well as the antibacterial drugs—Bactrim and Septra—can cause hives in those sensitive to sulfa. In addition, many vaginal creams, eyedrops (Ocusulf, Trusoft), acne medications (Sufacet-R, Klaron Lotion, Plexion Cleanser); burn preparations, such as Silvadine; cyclamates (Sucaryl, Sweeta, etc.); and most oral antidiabetic drugs, such as Diabinese, Orinase and Glucotrol, all contain sulfa!

Another common cause of hives is aspirin. Related to aspirin are other hive-producing chemicals known as salicylates. Salicylates appear in such products as root beer, wintergreen and mint flavorings, commercial bakery products, and mixes.

Certain food dyes and preservatives (such as sodium benzoate), insulin, and various vaccines to protect against measles and polio may also be common offenders. So is menthol, found in such diverse products as cigarettes, toothpastes, candies, jellies, Noxzema, room deodorants, lozenges, and shaving creams.

A list of medications that are apt to cause hives include the following:

## Trade/Brand-names

| | | |
|---|---|---|
| Abbokinase | Atarax | Claritin |
| Abilify | Atrovent | Codeine |
| Accolate | Avandia | Compazine |
| Accupril | Avapro | Copaxone |
| Aciphex | Avelox | Cosopt |
| Adalat | Avodart | Coumadin |
| Adderall | Azopt | Cozaar |
| Adipex-P | Azulfidine | Crestor |
| Aerobid | Bactrim | Cymbalta |
| Aggrastat | Benadryl | Darvon |
| Albenza | Benicar | Definity |
| Aldactone | Biaxin | Demerol |
| Alfenta | Biltricide | Denavir |
| Altace | Botox | Depen |
| Amaryl | Bumex | Desoxyn |
| Ambien | BuSpar | Diamox |
| Amevive | Caffeine | Didronel |
| Amoxil | Calan | Dimetane |
| Ampicillin | Campath | Dolobid |
| Anafranil | Capoten | Dolophine |
| Ansaid | Cardizem | Dramamine |
| Apresoline | Carafate | Dryvax |
| Arava | Casodex | Duragesic |
| Aricept | Catapres | Duricef |
| Arsenic | Ceclor | Dymelor |
| Asacol | Celebrex | DynaCirc |
| Aspirin | Chantix | Elavil |
| Atacand | Cialis | Eldepryl |

## Trade/Brand-names

| | | |
|---|---|---|
| Elidel | Levsinex | Norvir |
| Elmiron | Lipitor | Novahistine |
| Eloxatin | Lodine | Numorphan |
| Erythromycin | Lomotil | Oncaspar |
| Exelon | Lopid | Orencia |
| Fabrazyme | Lovenox | Orinase |
| Fansidar | Lozol | Orudis |
| Felbatol | Lunesta | Oxacillin |
| Feldene | Lupron | OxyContin |
| Femara | Luvox | Pamelor |
| Flagyl | Lyrica | Parnate |
| Flexeril | Macrobid | PEG-Intron |
| Flomax | Matulane | Penicillin |
| Floxin | Meridia | Pepcid |
| Fluoride | Mevacor | Phenergan |
| Forteo | Micardis | Plaquenil |
| Fosamax | Micronase | Plavix |
| Gabitril | Microsulfon | Plendil |
| Geodon | Minipress | Pravachol |
| Glucophage | Minocin | Precose |
| Glucotrol | Mobic | Prelone |
| Gris-PEG | Monodox | Prevacid |
| HCTZ | Monopril | Priftin |
| Humira | Motrin | Prilosec |
| Imodium | MS Contin | Procrit |
| Inderal | Mucomyst | Progesterone |
| Innohep | Nalfon | Prograf |
| Insulin | Namenda | Proleukin |
| Invirase | Navane | Prolixin |
| Keflex | Navelbine | Pronestyl |
| Kerlone | Neoral | Propylthiouracil |
| Ketek | Neulasta | Proscar |
| Lamictal | Nexavar | Protonix |
| Lamisil | Nexium | Proventil |
| Lanoxin | Nipent | Provera |
| Lasix | Norflex | Prozac |
| Lescol | Normozide | Pyrazinamide |
| Levaquin | Norvasc | Quinora |

## Trade/Brand-names

| | | |
|---|---|---|
| Q-Vel | Synercid | Vecuron |
| Reglan | Synthroid | Vesicare |
| Relafen | Talwin | Vicodin |
| Relenza | Tamiflu | Virazole |
| Remeron | Tasmar | Viread |
| Requip | Taxol | Vitamin B$_1$ |
| Rheumatrex | Tegretol | Vivactil |
| Rifadin | Testosterone | Voltaren |
| Risperdal | Thioplex | Wellbutrin |
| Ritalin | Ticlid | Xenical |
| Rituxan | Tobradex | Xifaxan |
| Robaxin | Tofranil | Xolair |
| Sabril | Tolectin | Xylocaine |
| Sandostatin | Tolinase | Xyrem |
| Seconal | Toprol | Zarontin |
| Septra | Toradol | Zestril |
| Serevent | Travatan | Zetia |
| Serzone | Trental | Zithromax |
| Sinemet | Tricor | Zocor |
| Singulair | Trileptal | Zofran |
| Soriatane | Trizivir | Zometa |
| Spiriva | Trobicin | Zomig |
| Sporanox | Tysabri | Zonegran |
| Starlix | Ultram | Zosyn |
| Strattera | Valtrex | Zovirax |
| Sufenta | Vancocin | Zyflo |
| Sular | Vasotec | Zyrtec |

# Itching

(Pruritus)

> Scratching is one of nature's sweetest
> gratifications of nature, and as ready at
> hand as any. —Michel de Montaigne

Itching, simply stated, is the urge to scratch. The medical term for itching is *pruritus*. It is a common, everyday experience ranging from a simple, fleeting annoyance (a mosquito bite) to the intense, distressing, unrelieved torment (the itch of scabies) that can result in sleepless nights.

Why do people itch? We know that the sensations of pain and itch are carried to the brain by the same nerve fibers, and we know that pain and itching points have similar distribution on the surface of the skin. We also know that it's possible, by varying the intensity of a stimulus (chemical, electrical, or physical) to cause either pain or itching on a certain portion of the skin.

Itching can thus be thought of as a sub-threshold pain, or, better still, as a pain that doesn't hurt. The difference, however, is that an itch occurs only in the skin; pain arises from deeper structures as well. And while itching leads to the urge to scratch, pain leads to withdrawal.

Have you ever bruised, scraped, or skinned your knee or elbow? Have you ever suffered from moderately severe sunburn? If you have, you may remember that at first there were varying degrees of pain. When the bruise, scrape, or burn began to heal, this pain was gradually transformed into an itch—a so-called "healing" itch: a peculiar sensation in the skin that produces a desire to scratch.

Commonly experienced, unpredictable, and poorly understood, itching is the symptom that most frequently prompts a person to visit a dermatologist. Different people experience, interpret, and tolerate itching in different degrees. One person's itch might be another person's tickle; one person's stinging itch can be another person's pain. If you have a high itch threshold, a transient mosquito bite or a brush with a poison ivy plant will rarely bother you. Less fortunate people will itch unmercifully at the least provocation, such as a mild allergy to nickel earrings or a simple rash from a leather watchband. No one knows why.

More frequently than not, generalized drug-induced itching without any visible signs is one of the least common adverse reactions to drugs. Many years ago, scientists thought that the basic cause of itching was the release of a chemical substance called histamine. We now know that itching can be caused by a breakdown of various tissue proteins, and can be precipitated by a variety of stimuli such as the following:

- Athlete's foot
- Blood disorders
- Chemicals
- Cold sores
- Cosmetics
- Foods (berries, seafood, nuts)
- Hodgkin's disease
- Impetigo
- Infestations: lice, mites (scabies)
- Insect bites and stings
- Leukemias
- Medications (see list on page 131)
- Metals (nickel, chromium)
- Paints and sprays
- Physical: heat, cold, pressure, and friction
- Plants (poison ivy)
- Psychogenic: anxiety, tension, and emotional stress
- Skin disorders: eczema, allergy rashes, hives, lichen planus, dry skin
- Systemic disease: diabetes and other hormonal disorders, liver and kidney problems, malignant diseases

Medications that have been reported to cause itching include the following:

## Trade/Brand-names

| | | |
|---|---|---|
| Abbokinase | Aredia | Celestone |
| Abilify | Aricept | Celexa |
| Accolate | Arimidex | CellCept |
| Accupril | Arsenic | Celontin |
| Accutane | Asacol | Cerebyx |
| Aceon | Aspirin | Cerezyme |
| Achromycin | Astelin | Cerubidine |
| Aciphex | Atacand | Chemet |
| Actifed | Atarax | Cialis |
| Actigall | Atrovent | Cipro |
| Actonel | Avandia | Clarinex |
| Adalat | Avapro | Claritin |
| Adriamycin | Avelox | Cleocin |
| Aerobid | Avodart | Clinoril |
| Aggrenox | Axert | Clomid |
| Agrylin | Axid | Cocaine |
| Aleve | Azactam | Copaxone |
| Alina | Azulfidine | Cordarone |
| Alkeran | Bactrim | Cosopt |
| Allegra | Beconase | Coumadin |
| Alphagan | Benecid | Cozaar |
| Altace | Benicar | Crixivan |
| Amaryl | Betapace | Cubicin |
| Ambien | Bexxar | Cymbalta |
| Amevive | Bismuth | Cytadren |
| Amicar | Blenoxane | Cytosar |
| Amoxil | Botox | Cytovene |
| Anafranil | Brevibloc | Dacogen |
| Ancobon | Bumex | Dantrolene |
| Andro-LA | Campath | Daypro |
| Ansaid | Campral | Decadron |
| Anthrax vaccine | Capoten | Depakene |
| Anzamet | Carafate | Depakote |
| Apresoline | Cardizem | Depen |
| Aptivus | Cardura | Desferal |
| Aralen | Casodex | Diabinese |
| Aransep | Catapres | Didronel |
| Arava | Celebrex | Dimetane |

## Trade/Brand-names

| | | |
|---|---|---|
| Diovan | Flexeril | Intron-A |
| Dipentum | Flomax | Invanz |
| Diprivan | Flonase | Invirase |
| Ditropan | Floxin | Iopidine |
| Dolobid | Fludara | Iressa |
| Dolophine | Flurazepam | Keflex |
| Dopram | Forteo | Keppra |
| Doral | Fosamax | Ketek |
| Dostinex | Foscavir | Lamisil |
| Duragesic | Fragmin | Lanoxin |
| Duricef | Frisium | Lariam |
| DynaCirc | Fucidin | Lasix |
| Effexor | Fungizone | Lescol |
| Eldepryl | Fuzeon | Leustatin |
| Elestat | Gabitril | Levaquin |
| Elmiron | Gastrocrom | Levitra |
| Elspar | Gastrografin | Lexapro |
| Emcyt | Gemzar | Lincocin |
| Emtriva | Gleevec | Lipitor |
| Enablex | Glucotrol | Lodine |
| Enbrel | Glucovance | Lomotil |
| Eraxis | Gold | Loniten |
| Erbitux | Haldol | Lopid |
| Erythromycin | Hectorol | Lorabid |
| Estrogens | Hepsera | Lotensin |
| Ethyol | Herceptin | Lovenox |
| Eulexin | Hexalen | Loxitane |
| Evoxin | Hivid | Lozol |
| Exelon | Hycamtin | Lumigan |
| Exovac | Hyperstat | Lunesta |
| Extraneal | Hyzaar | Lupron |
| Factive | Imdur | Lyrica |
| Famvir | Imitrex | Macrobid |
| Fareston | Imodium | Malarone |
| Felbatol | Inapsine | Matulane |
| Femara | Inderal | Mavik |
| Fiorinal | Indocin | Maxair |
| Flagyl | Innohep | Maxalt |

## Trade/Brand-names

| | | |
|---|---|---|
| Meridia | Orencia | Relafen |
| Methadone | Orfadin | Relpax |
| Mevacor | Orinase | Remeron |
| Micardis | Ornidyl | Remicade |
| Minipress | Orudis | Remodulin |
| Minocin | Oxsoralen | ReoPro |
| Moban | OxyContin | Revlimid |
| Mobic | Panretin | Reyataz |
| Monopril | Paraplatin | Rhinocort |
| Monurol | Parnate | Rifadin |
| Morphine | Patanol | Rilutek |
| MS Contin | Paxil | Rituxan |
| Mucomyst | PEG-Intron | Robaxin |
| Myambutol | Pepcid | Robinul |
| Myleran | Plavix | Rythmol |
| Mylotarg | Pletal | Salagen |
| Namenda | Pravachol | Sandostatin |
| Nardil | Prevacid | Sectral |
| Natrecor | Prialt | Seroquel |
| Navane | Priftin | Serpasil |
| Navelbine | Prilosec | Serzone |
| Nebilet | Primaquine | Simulect |
| Neoral | Primaxin | Sinemet |
| Neupro | Proamatine | Sinequan |
| Neurontin | Procrit | Singulair |
| Neutrexin | Progesterone | Skelaxin |
| Nexavar | Prograf | Skelid |
| Nexium | Proleukin | Sonata |
| Nipent | Pronestyl | Soriatane |
| Nizoral | Propylthiouracil | Spiriva |
| Nolvadex | Proscar | Sporanox |
| Normozide | ProSom | SPRYCEL |
| Noroxin | Protonix | Stadol |
| Norpace | Provera | Starlix |
| Norvasc | Prozac | Strattera |
| Novahistine | Quinora | Stromectol |
| Nubain | Q-Vel | Suboxone |
| Ontak | Rapamune | Sufenta |

## Trade/Brand-names

| | | |
|---|---|---|
| Sular | Travatan | Wellbutrin |
| Sustiva | Trelstar | Xanax |
| Symmetrel | Trental | Xeloda |
| Synarel | Triasox | Xenical |
| Synercid | Tricor | Xibrom |
| Synthroid | Trizivir | Xifaxan |
| Talwin | Trobicin | Xolair |
| Tambocor | Tysabri | Xylocaine |
| Tapazole | Ultracet | Xyrem |
| Tarceva | Ultram | Xyzal |
| Targretin | Ultravist | Zarontin |
| Tarka | Valstar | Zaroxolyn |
| Tasmar | Valtrex | Zelnorm |
| Taxol | Vantas | Zenapax |
| Taxotere | Vascase | Zevalin |
| Tegretol | Vasotec | Ziac |
| Temodar | Velcade | Zithromax |
| Tenex | VePesid | Zocor |
| Testosterone | Vesicare | Zofran |
| Tetracycline | Vfend | Zolinza |
| Teveten | Vicodin | Zometa |
| Thalidomid | Vidaza | Zomig |
| Thioplex | Videx | Zonegran |
| Ticar | Viracept | Zostavax |
| Ticlid | Virazole | Zosyn |
| Tolinase | Viread | Zovirax |
| Tonocard | Visken | Zyban |
| Topamax | Vistaril | Zyflo |
| Toprol | Vitamin $B_1$ | Zyrtec |
| Toradol | Vitamin $B_3$ | Zyvox |
| Tracleer | Voltaren | |

## Lupus Erythematosus (LE)

> The wolf, I'm afraid, is inside tearing up
> the place. I've been in the hospital 50
> days already this year.
> —Flannery O'Connor, a few days be-
> fore succumbing to her progressive and
> inexorable fatal lupus.

Lupus erythematosus (also lupus or LE) is one of those curious diseases that can masquerade as any of a dozen other
medical maladies. Its variety of symptoms include fever, chills,
headache, weakness, fatigue, hair loss, joint pains, chest
pains, epileptic seizures, personality changes, and rashes.
Any or all of these symptoms may be part of this complicated
disease we commonly call LE.

The term *lupus* (Latin for "wolf") is attributed to the thirteenth-
century physician Rogerius who used it to describe erosive
(eaten away) facial lesions that were reminiscent of a wolf's
bite. Classical descriptions of the various skin features of lupus
were made in the early nineteenth century.

LE is a chronic inflammation of connective tissue—the so-
called body "glue"—that binds our cells together. As such, it
is considered a connective tissue, or collagen, disease and
is often classified in the rheumatic group of diseases along
with rheumatic fever and rheumatoid arthritis. Every part of our
bodies—all our organs, our muscles, blood, joints, skin—has
this connective tissue, and thus may be affected by LE.

No one really knows what causes LE. This puzzling condition, which affects over 500,000 people in the United States,
is most likely due to an "autoimmune process"—a technical
way of saying that the body, due to some unexplained allergy,
produces certain abnormal substances called autoantibodies
that attack and destroy its own tissues. Normally, when foreign substances (antigens) such as disease-producing germs
or allergens attack your body, it responds by producing anti-

bodies to fight off these harmful invaders. In people with LE, this normal defense mechanism breaks down. And instead of attacking the antigens, the antibodies attack the body's own tissues.

It is important to know there are two types of LE. One is the benign or "friendly" type, called the *discoid* variety of LE. Triggered by some external factor, such as sunlight or injury, discoid LE shows up as red, scaly patches symmetrically distributed over the sun-exposed areas of the body—the "butterfly" areas—the cheeks, nose, ears, scalp, backs of the hands, and occasionally the "V" of the neck. The patches of LE can also affect the beard and scalp, usually resulting in permanent hair loss.

These patches grow larger over a period of months or years, forming disc-shaped (discoid) patches. They slowly lose their reddish color and become white and depressed. This depression—essentially a scar—is the end result of a typical discoid lesion.

Discoid LE affects all races, is more common in young adults, and occurs twice as often in women as in men. If you have discoid LE, it's important to see a dermatologist. While the condition itself is relatively harmless, these "discs" may be harbingers of some underlying condition that can flare up into systemic lupus erythematosus (SLE).

SLE is a serious variety of LE that can affect and damage any or all of the body's organs or systems including the kidneys, liver, heart, lungs, bone marrow, and joints. Fortunately, only about one in ten people with discoid LE ever progress to the systemic or internal type of the disease.

One of the triggering mechanisms that may convert the "friendly" condition into the more serious, "unfriendly" variety is sun exposure. People with LE must strictly avoid the beaches, sunbathing in general, and tropical cruises.

Other factors can turn the "benign" form of the disease into the more serious type:

• Certain medications (see list on page 137)

- Fatigue
- Injury
- Overwork
- Stress

Some well-known celebrities afflicted by lupus include the following:
- Charles Kuralt (died of lupus in 1997)
- Ferdinand Marcos (died of lupus in 1989)
- Flannery O'Connor (died of lupus in 1964)
- J Dilla (died of lupus in 2006)
- Louisa May Alcott
- Michael Jackson
- Ray Walston
- Tim Raines

Medications that have been reported to cause or aggravate lupus include the following:

## Trade/Brand-names

| | | |
|---|---|---|
| Anafranil | HCTZ | Septra |
| Anthrax vaccine | Humira | SPRYCEL |
| Asacol | Intron A | Taxotere |
| Bactrim | Lamisil | Thelin |
| Capoten | Lasix | Ticlid |
| Cardura | Lescol | Trilafon |
| Celontin | Lipitor | Trileptal |
| Copaxone | Mevacor | Vasotec |
| Cosopt | Minipress | Vfend |
| Dapsone | Minocin | Virazole |
| Declomycin | Normozide | Zarontin |
| Dilantin | PEG-Intron | Zestril |
| Diuril | Pravachol | Zocor |
| Exovac | Rythmol | Zonegran |
| Gastrocrom | Sectral | |

## Psoriasis

> Each morning, I vacuum my bed. My
> torture is skin deep: there is no pain,
> not even itching; we lepers live a long
> time, and are ironically healthy in other
> respects. Lusty, though we are loath-
> some to love. Keen-sighted, though we
> hate to look upon ourselves. The name
> of the disease, spiritually speaking, is
> Humiliation.
> —John Updike. From the *Journal of a
> Leper. The New Yorker*, July 19, 1986,
> 28–33.

Psoriasis is a stubborn, chronic, and as yet incurable disease of the skin. Some eight million people—150,000 new cases annually—suffer from psoriasis in the United States alone. And they spend more than $1 billion a year ($2,000 every minute!) to treat this poorly understood ailment.

Psoriasis—the word comes from the Greek *psora*, which means "itch"—was considered a form of leprosy in biblical times. But this "disease of healthy people" doesn't threaten or shorten lives. It is neither an infection nor an allergy. It probably is not due to any vitamin or mineral deficiency. It doesn't leave scars or make you lose your hair. And, except in severe cases, it doesn't interfere with physical activities. (In fact, it may not even itch.) To the psoriasis sufferer, however, it can be an emotionally disabling and traumatic disorder leading to considerable psychological difficulties, functional declines, disruption of lifestyle, interpersonal problems, and, consequently, a diminished quality of life. One study found that almost a quarter of psoriasis patients have contemplated suicide because of their inability to cope with the disease.

Patches of raised, red skin covered by silvery-white scales characterize psoriasis. It can occur at any age but commonly begins in young adulthood. The natural history of psoriasis is marked by frequent flares and remissions. It usually recurs at unpredictable intervals and may be worse in the winter. It is often precipitated or aggravated by physical or emotional stress, upper respiratory infections, strep throat, viral infections, AIDS, alcoholic beverages, obesity, certain oral medications (lithium, beta-blockers, ACE-inhibitors, and anti-malarial drugs are but a few), and skin injuries such as scratches, cuts, and burns, including sunburn.

Psoriasis is not contagious. It does seem to run in families—about one-third of psoriatic patients have a family history of the condition—although the pattern of heredity is not clear. If, however, both your parents have psoriasis, the chances are fifty-fifty that you, too, will inherit it. Psoriasis is also associated with a form of arthritis that affects the joints of the fingers. Up to 30 percent of people with psoriasis have symptoms of arthritis.

No one knows the cause of psoriasis, but we do know how it comes about. Normal skin cells have a life span of about twenty-eight days. This is the time it takes for a cell to be born, move to the outer surface of the skin, and flake off.

In psoriasis, this orderly process goes awry due to some abnormality in the mechanism that makes the skin grow and replace itself. The skin cells develop, reproduce, and die at a rate ten times faster than the normal cells, causing a buildup of scales in thick and sharply bordered patches. These layers of dead skin form silvery-looking plaques that are shed in clumps, leaving the skin beneath red and sore-looking. These patches may be small—the size of a matchhead or smaller—or extremely large, covering the entire body; if they appear in the body's creases and folds, they may cause itching and pain. Although psoriasis can affect any part of the skin, the patches usually occur on the elbows, knees, and scalp.

Psoriasis comes in many shapes and forms. It can, for example, limit itself to the fingernails and toenails as small pits or stippling or loosening of the nails from their beds. Sometimes it affects the genital area and can limit sexual activity. In extreme cases, it is widespread, with painful cracks and total body redness and scaling, causing severe embarrassment. This, in turn, can lead to psychological problems: the true "heartbreak" of psoriasis.

Psoriasis is one of the most difficult of all chronic skin disorders to manage. Therapies that seem to be successful can suddenly stop being effective. Psoriasis can go into spontaneous remission and disappear only to reappear just as abruptly.

Celebrities past and present with psoriasis:

- Admiral Bull Halsey
- Art Garfunkel
- Benjamin Franklin
- Carrie Dee English
- Dennis Hopper
- Ernest Hemingway
- Jerry Mathers
- John Updike
- Joseph Stalin
- Vladimir Nabokov

Medications that are known to cause or aggravate psoriasis include the following:

## Trade/Brand-names

| | | |
|---|---|---|
| Abilify | Amoxil | Bactrim |
| Aceon | Anafranil | BCG vaccine |
| Aciphex | Androgel | Betapace |
| Actigall | Android | Biaxin |
| Adriamycin | Android-F | Botulinum toxin |
| Advil | Androstenedione | Brevibloc |
| Aggrenox | Arsenic | Capoten |
| Aldara | Asacol | Cardizem |
| Allegra | Aspirin | Carteol |
| Altace | Atacand | Catapres |
| Amaryl | Augmentin | Celebrex |
| Amevive | Azulfidine | Celestone |

## Trade/Brand-names

Celexa
Chantix
Cognex
Copaxone
Cordarone
Coreg
Corgard
Cytadren
Cytovene
Depakote
Depen
Desyrel
Diamox
Diovan
Ecstacy
Effexor
Efudex
Enbrel
Exelon
Femara
Flonase
Foscavir
Gabitril
Gleevec
Glucotrol
Gold
Humira
Hydrea
Hygroton
Inderal
Indocin
Intron-A

Inverase
Kerlone
Lamisil
Lanoxin
Lariam
Leukeran
Levatol
Lithobid
Lopid
Methicillin
Methotrexate
Micronase
Mobic
Monodox
Morphine
Nebilet
Neoral
Neupogen
Nipent
Normozide
Norvir
Oral contraceptives
Orudis
Paxil
Pediazole
PEG-Intron
Plaquenil
Plavix
Prelone
Prilosec
Principen
Proleukin

Provigil
Prozac
Quinora
Q-Vel
Raptiva
Rebetron
Relpax
Remicade
Requip
Risperdal
Sectral
Septra
Soriatane
SSKI
Sumycin
Tagamet
Tambocor
Tegretol
Tenormin
Timoptic
Toprol
Trileptal
Vasotec
Vfend
Visken
Voltaren
Wellbutrin
Zantac
Ziac
Zyban
Zyprexa

Note: It is interesting that several of the newer biologic response modifiers that are being used to treat psoriasis such as Humira, Remicade, Amevive, Raptiva, and Enbrel can also cause and/or aggravate psoriasis.

## Pigmentation

Normal skin color is dependent upon the amount and size of certain pigment granules in the upper layers of the skin. This basic skin color is determined at birth and cannot be altered. Human skin color can range from almost black to nearly color-less (appearing pinkish white due to the blood in the skin) in different people. Skin color is determined by the amount and type of melanin, the pigment in the skin. As a general pattern, people with ancestors from tropical regions (with greater sun-light exposure) have darker skin than people with ancestors from subtropical regions, but this is far from a hard-and-fast rule.

All human skin contains three important pigments:

1. *Melanin*: This black pigment in your skin is produced by special pigment cells called *melanocytes*. All of us have the same number of these melanocytes in our skin (approximately 60,000 per square inch).

Racial and ethnic variations in skin color depend on the size and shape of these melanocytes, the amount of melanin they produce, the speed at which the pigment is formed, the manner in which this pigment is concentrated in the skin, and the color of the melanin, which can vary from light tan to black.

Melanin is produced in the skin as small, insoluble gran-ules. Where there are no melanin granules, the skin is white; the more melanin granules, the darker the skin. The variations in your particular skin color—tan, brown, black—will depend upon the concentration of these granules in your epidermis.

In black people, melanin production is evenly distributed, producing uniform skin color. In redheads, and in some blonds with blue eyes, melanin is produced in clumps, resulting in splotchy pigmentation or freckles. Freckles, probably the most common pigmentary alteration in the skin, first appear in chil-dren at about the age of six as flat, light brown, pigmented spots over sun-exposed skin. During the summer, they have a tendency to increase in number, size, and darkness.

The depth of the melanin granules will also affect the color of your skin: the deeper the granules, the more your skin will take on a bluish cast.

2. *Hemoglobin*: This pigment is responsible for giving red blood cells their color. If you are anemic, your skin will be pale; if you have too much hemoglobin, your skin will take on a ruddy complexion.

3. *Carotene*: This pigment, which gives your skin a yellowish cast, comes from outside the body and is dependent upon what you eat. A diet consisting of large amounts of oranges, carrots, and squash can be responsible for an orange-yellow staining of the skin.

## Excessive Pigmentation

The most common cause of excessive pigmentation is an increased stimulation in the production of melanin due to certain hormonal changes, sun exposure, or a combination of the two. This condition, called *melasma*, appears as a dark, splotchy, brownish pigmentation on the face that develops slowly and fades with time. It usually affects women but occasionally is seen in young men who use aftershave lotions, scented soaps, and other toiletries.

*Melasma* is especially common in young white women, who often develop this blotchiness on their foreheads, cheeks, and mustache areas. It occurs frequently during pregnancy and is more common in brunettes than in blondes. Often called "the mask of pregnancy," melasma is more pronounced in summer due to sun exposure, and usually fades a few months after delivery. Repeated pregnancies, however, often increase the intensity of this pigmentation.

Melasma also occurs as a side effect of taking the higher-dose birth control pills. It may also be noted in apparently healthy, normal, nonpregnant women due to some mild and harmless hormonal imbalance.

Sun exposure, following the use of deodorant soaps, scented toiletries, and various cosmetics, can also produce this mottled pigmentation. This is called a *phototoxic reaction*; it is due to ultraviolet radiation being absorbed by the chemical substance (perfume, cologne, and other types of fragrance) on the skin. This pigmentation often extends down to the sun-exposed areas of the neck and may be more pronounced on the left side of the forehead, face, and neck due to sun exposure while driving a car (in the United States).

Excess pigmentation can also be triggered by injury to the skin (burns, abrasions, bruises), by inflammatory disorders of the skin particularly in dark-skinned people (acne, eczema, contact dermatitis, pityriasis rosea, lichen planus), by X-rays, and by heat.

Drug-induced pigmentation represents 10 to 20 percent of all cases of acquired hyperpigmentation. Some of the drugs implicated in hyperpigmentation include the following:

## Trade/Brand-names

| | | |
|---|---|---|
| Accutane | Fansidar | Oxsoralen |
| Adriamycin | Halog | Phenergan |
| Aldara | Hydrea | Plaquenil |
| Arsenic | Ifex | Prednisone |
| Blenoxane | Inapsine | Prolixin |
| Catapres | Leukeran | Pyridium |
| Cerubidine | Levulan | Quinora |
| Cipro | Lodine | Rescula |
| Compazine | Loniten | Rheumatrex |
| Cortisone | Lumigan | Sumycin |
| Cosmegen | Lupron | Sutent |
| Crixivan | Matulane | Tapazole |
| Decadron | Minocin | Taxol |
| Declomycin | Moban | Taxotere |
| Duragesic | Monodox | Tegretol |
| Efudex | Mustargen | Thioplex |
| Ellence | Myleran | Thorazine |
| Emtriva | Neoral | Travatan |

## Trade/Brand-names

| | | |
|---|---|---|
| Trizivir | Videx | Xylocaine |
| VePesid | Vitamin B3 | |
| Vidaza | Xalatan | |

## Sweating

(Perspiration, Diaphoresis)

> It is not manly to fear sweat.
> —Seneca, *Moral Epistles to Lucilius*,
> XXXI, vii, 31

All normal, healthy people sweat. Some more, some less. And all healthy people smell when they sweat. This, too, is normal.

Sweat is important in regulating body temperature. Despite enormous changes in the temperature of our external environment—be it tropical or subzero—our internal body temperature remains fairly constant.

When you are exposed to excessive heat, the sweat glands pour out their watery secretion (sweat) and carry out the vital task of cooling your body. This thermoregulatory mechanism has allowed us to adapt to the hottest climates.

Sweat is composed of the secretion of two types of glands: the two million eccrine glands distributed over the entire body, and the localized apocrine glands, which are restricted primarily to the armpits, the anogenital region, and the nipples. The growth of the apocrine glands is regulated by a hormone that begins to form about the time of puberty and decreases markedly in old age. (This is why children under the age of twelve and elderly people do not suffer from "body odor.") These apocrine glands become active after puberty, respond to hormonal secretions, and are stimulated by emotional factors such as stress and sexual excitement.

Sweat itself is essentially odorless. Most of the odor is due to the action of various bacteria on the milky secretion of the apocrine sweat glands. These bacteria are most active in moist and warm environments, particularly hairy armpits.

Sweat from body regions devoid of apocrine glands can also have an unpleasant odor. For example, the odor of certain aromatic foods and spices (such as garlic and onions) are secreted in eccrine sweat. And eccrine sweat from prolonged exercising can cause an unpleasant odor due to bacterial action on the soft, wet skin. This is the most common cause of foot odor.

Normally, we lose about two quarts of liquid through perspiration each day. Perspiration is not voluntary. You cannot decide when you want to perspire, and you cannot tell yourself to stop this mechanism. Emotional and environmental factors (heat) influence the degree of sweating, especially over the palms, soles, armpits, and forehead. Cigarette smoking may also be responsible for excessive perspiration. You can, however, "harness" this mechanism somewhat by using antiperspirants and deodorants.

Antiperspirants are compounds that reduce the volume of perspiration. Deodorants are products used to mask, diminish, or prevent perspiration odor.

Perspiration (also called *diaphoresis*, sweating, or sometimes *transpiration*) is the production and evaporation of a fluid, consisting primarily of water as well as a smaller amount of *sodium chloride* (the main constituent of "table salt"), that is excreted by the sweat glands in the skin of mammals. In humans, sweating is primarily a means of *thermoregulation*, although it has been proposed that components of male sweat can act as *pheromonal* cues. Evaporation of sweat from the skin surface has a cooling effect due to the *latent heat* of evaporation of water. Hence, in hot weather, or when the individual's muscles heat up due to exertion, more sweat is produced. Sweating is increased by nervousness and nausea and decreased by cold. Animals with few sweat glands, such as dogs, accomplish similar temperature regulation results by panting, which evaporates water from the moist lining of the oral cavity, especially the tongue.

Medications that have been reported to cause sweating include the following:

### Trade/Brand-names

| | | |
|---|---|---|
| Actos | Focalin | Ritalin |
| Adrenaline | Gleevec | Rituxan |
| Adriamycin | Glucotrol | Robinul |
| Alomide | Hivid | Rynatuss |
| Amaryl | Imdur | Sinemet |
| Amitiza | Indocin | Starlix |
| Aricept | Insulin | Streptomycin |
| Arsenic | Isordil | Synthroid |
| Aspirin | Lanvis | Tagamet |
| Atacand | Levsinex | Tensilon |
| Avandia | Librax | Thyroid |
| Bentyl | Lithobid | Tolinase |
| Botox | Matulane | Topamax |
| Celexa | Methadone | Trexan |
| Cerubidine | Micronase | Trizivir |
| Clozaril | Narcan | Tygacil |
| Cognex | Neoral | Tylenol |
| Copaxone | Nexium | Tysabri |
| Cordarone | Nicotine | Ultracet |
| Coreg | Novantrone | Ultram |
| Cymbalta | Orinase | Urecholine |
| Cytomel | Parnate | Vantas |
| Diabinese | Prandin | Vesicare |
| Diamox | Prevacid | Vidaza |
| Ditropan | Prezista | Xyrem |
| Dopram | Priftin | Zenapax |
| Exelon | Progesterone | Zonegran |
| Exovac | Reminyl | Zyrtec |
| Femara | Revlimid | |
| Flagyl | Rifadin | |

## Hyperhidrosis

(Excessive Sweating)

Hyperhidrosis is the name given to excessive and uncontrollable sweating. It is the condition characterized by abnormally increased perspiration, in excess of that required for regulation of body temperature. Usually beginning in either childhood or adolescence, hyperhydrosis can affect any site on the body. The sites most commonly affected are the palms, soles, armpits, and groins as a result of the relatively high concentration of sweat glands in these areas. The cause may be unknown, or it may be secondary to other diseases, metabolic disorders, fevers, or medication use. Hyperhidrosis exists in three forms: emotionally induced (in which it affects the palms, soles, and armpits), localized, or generalized. Hyperhidrosis affects millions of people around the world and, according to some studies, about 3 percent of the population.

Normal sweating—also known as *diaphoresis*—is essential to keep the body cool; it should not interfere with the ability to interact and function. Hyperhidrosis can impact the means to carry out routine everyday jobs and may even be an occupational risk. Anxiety can exacerbate the situation for many sufferers. A common complaint is that sufferers get nervous because they sweat; they then sweat more because they are nervous. Patients afflicted with hyperhidrosis often experience embarrassment and frustration and a reduction in the quality of their life.

Excessive sweating of the hands interferes with many routine activities, such as securely grasping objects. Some hyperhidrosis sufferers avoid situations where they will come into physical contact with others, such as greeting a person with a handshake. Excess sweat on the hands may soil paper and artwork and make it virtually impossible to play many musical instruments. People with hyperhidrosis may find it impossible to pursue careers in fields that require contact with paper, metal, or electrical devices. Sweaty feet develop an unpleasant smell, ruin footwear, and are prone to *dermatitis,* ringworm, or secondary infection.

Generalized hyperhidrosis may be secondary to numerous conditions including the following:

- Cardiovascular disorders
- Chronic alcoholism and withdrawal (Excessive sweating of the palms and soles is observed in persons with chronic alcoholism.)
- Febrile illnesses
- Heat, humidity, exercise
- Hodgkin's disease
- Malignant tumors
- Medications (see list below)
- Menopause
- Metabolic disorders (thyroid illness, diabetes, hypoglycemia, gout)
- Neurologic diseases
- Obesity
- Parkinsonism
- Shock
- Tuberculosis (causes night sweats)

Generalized hyperhidrosis usually begins in adulthood, and the sweating occurs during both waking and sleeping. Such cases require investigation of potential underlying causes, such as medications and systemic illnesses.

Medications that may cause excessive sweating include the following:

### Trade/Brand-names

| | | |
|---|---|---|
| Aleve | Celexa | Imitrex |
| Amitzia | Chantix | Marplan |
| Aromasin | Duragesic | Monopril |
| Botox | DynaCirc | Naprosyn |
| Butisol | Effexor | Nexium |
| Capoten | Hepatitis A Vaccine | Noroxin |

## Body Odor

(Bromhidrosis)

Body odor or bromhidrosis (also called *bromidrosis*, *osmidrosis*, and *ozochrotia*) is the offensive smell caused by the combination of perspiration (sweat), bacteria and fungi always present on the skin. While sweat itself is typically an odorless body secretion, these organisms proliferate rapidly in the presence of sweat and decompose these secretions. The resulting by-products of this breakdown have a strong disagreeable odor.

Everyone sweats. The secretion of sweat is an essential function of the skin for temperature regulation and water metabolism. The body has two types of sweat glands, and both types produce sweat that is made up mainly of water. The eccrine glands, which are located on almost every portion of the body, manufacture the sweat that cools the body. The apocrine glands, which evolve during puberty, and are thought to serve a biological role in sexual attraction, and contain a significant amount of organic matter, including pheromone hormones. These apocrine glands are found in the armpits, around the nipples, and in the groin area, and they produce sweat that can make you reek.

As a rule, the human body has a slight sweaty or musky odor. Here are some tips for preventing body odor:

• Bathe regularly. Daily bathing with soap and water, and using deodorants or antiperspirants, is enough to prevent a truly objectionable, noxious odor. Nothing beats personal cleanliness for eliminating odors.

- Keep clothing clean. Clothing collects not only the odors but also the germs responsible for them.
- Wear only cotton shirts and blouses. Polyester fibers do not "breathe," and they often retain odor even after laundering.
- Shave your armpits regularly. Bacteria *love* armpits.
- Avoid garlic, onions, and asparagus. These can produce offensive odors, especially in the summertime.
- Cut down on caffeine (coffee, tea, and cola drinks), which stimulates sweat gland activity.

There are several factors that may contribute to chronic body odor:
- Anxiety and stress which stimulate perspiration
- Cancer, hemorrhoids, and ulcers which may produce offensive foul discharges on the skin
- Chain-smoking and heavy drinking (Nicotine and alcohol increase the rate of perspiration and are excreted through the skin and lungs.)
- Ingestion of coffee and other stimulants which increase apocrine gland secretion
- Disorders such as liver disease, kidney disease, diabetes, yeast, and fungal infections
- Foods such as garlic, onions, spicy food, alcohol
- Gastrointestinal ailments such as GERD (acid reflux)
- Hyperhidrosis or excessive sweating
- Imbalance in the bacteria inhabiting the alimentary canal, sometimes due to antibiotics
- Inability to digest particular foods (Undigested foods cause the body to give off disagreeable smells.)
- Poor hygiene and inadequate bathing
- The aging process (Aging causes functional changes in cells. The rate at which cells multiply tends to slow down as we age, and certain cells

that are important for our immune system to work
properly also decrease with age.)
- *Trimethylaminuria*, a hereditary condition that calls
  for avoiding fish and other dietary sources of choline
- Vaginal infections caused by bacteria called
  Gardnerella

Despite some unpleasant side effects, sweating is in fact
an essential part of keeping your body cool. For most people,
however, sweating itself is a minor nuisance. The odor that
sometimes occurs when you sweat is probably more troublesome. If you find this offensive, you're not alone—Americans
spend $2 billion a year on antiperspirants and deodorants.

In some cultures, intense body odor is considered a desir-
able quality, suggestive of greater sexual attractiveness and
prowess. In the United States, however, a pungent body odor
is not going to make you the life of the party. So compelling is
our cultural distaste for body odor that every day practically
all Americans over the age of twelve reach for one product or
another that will allow them to feel comfortable and secure in
the company of others.

In 1919, Odo-Ro-No was the first company to use the term
"B.O.," indicating "body odor." An advertisement for their deodorant, aimed at women, directed potential customers to take
the "Armhole Odor Test" and counseled them that social success hinged on eradicating "B.O."

Ages ago, when humans lived in caves, they were less anx-
ious about body odor. They must have reeked. Anthropologists
believe that this funkiness helped keep early man from being
some predator's feast—or snack. The scent was so rank that
the creature about to eat them would practically recoil in disgust at the smell and would move on to eat something less
nauseating. As in the case of the skunk, putrid body odor is a
marvelous defense mechanism.

The ancient Egyptians, when not constructing pyramids,
were working hard at concealing their own stench. They in-

vented a sweet-smelling aromatic bath and applied perfume to their armpits. Women placed globs of scented wax on their heads that gradually softened and melted throughout the day, spreading the delightful scent as well as camouflaging the offensive.

The ancient Greeks regularly bathed in and drenched themselves with perfume. The early Romans took baths in perfume, soaked their clothes in it, and doused their horses and pets in it.

In the Middle Ages, when the Church resolved that being naked was evil—even in the bath—people all but stopped cleaning themselves. Those with the money for it tried to cover the stench by using perfume, a habit that persists even to this day.

In 1888, Mum, a waxy cream deodorant for the armpits was developed. It was difficult to apply, extremely messy to use, and almost impossible to wash off. A few years later, Everdry, the first antiperspirant to use aluminum chloride, evolved. Both products were yucky, took hours to dry, and, in addition to stinging, ate through clothing. In 1952, Ban, the first roll-on was marketed and, in the early 1960s, Right Guard, the first aerosol, was introduced.

No antiperspirant completely stops the flow of perspiration. It would be undesirable if the flow was entirely stopped, because secretion of sweat is an essential function of the skin for temperature regulation and water metabolism.

A note about the differences between antiperspirants and deodorants: Antiperspirants are compounds that reduce the volume of perspiration. Deodorants are products used to mask, diminish, or prevent perspiration odor. Deodorants that do not claim to check perspiration are classified as cosmetics. If the same preparation is labeled an "antiperspirant," it becomes a drug, as it alleges to change a bodily function, and therefore requires a prescription from a doctor.

## Trivia:

The loss of sexual appetite because your partner has wicked B.O. is known as *ozoamblyrosis*.

Henry IV, the king of France from 1589–1610, was a victim of bromidrosis. Proximity to him was insufferable to his mistresses and to his courtiers who said that his odor was like that of decaying flesh.

The seventeenth-century French writer, Tallemant, averred that when his wife, Marie de Medicis, approached the bridal night with him, she perfumed her apartments and her person with the essences of the flowers of her country in order that she might be spared the foul-smelling odor of her spouse.

In 2007, *Maxim* released the following list of smelly celebrities. The same list brought Britney Spears to tears after she was named on it.

- Amy Winehouse
- Andy Rooney
- Billy Joel
- Cisco Adler
- Dennis Franz
- Flavor Flav
- John Madden
- Louie Anderson
- Mark Boone Jr.
- Meat Loaf
- Nick Nolte
- Paul Giamatti
- Pete Doherty
- Rob Schneider
- Steve Buscemi
- Woody Allen

A variety of medications has been reported to cause body odor. The nine drugs below, and many others, may be responsible for the excretion of odors:

## Trade/Brand-names

| | | |
|---|---|---|
| Felbatol | Omega-3-Acids | Selenium |
| Levocarnitine | Provera | Synarel |
| Lupron | Salagen | Topamax |

# Chapter 2:  Hair

## Hair Loss

(Alopecia)

Many drugs have been reported to cause hair loss. Commonly appearing as a *diffuse alopecia*, hair loss affects women much more frequently than men and is limited in most instances to the scalp. Axillary and pubic hairs are rarely affected, except with anticoagulants.

The hair loss from agents that suppress cellular growth and multiplication, also known as *chemotherapeutic* or *cytostatic agents*, begins about two weeks after the onset of therapy. It is a result of the interruption of the growing cycle of hair. With other drugs, such as cholesterol-lowering pills, the hair loss does not begin until two to five months after the medication has been begun. The scalp is normal, and the drug-induced alopecia is almost always reversible within one to three months after the therapy has been discontinued. The regrown hair is frequently depigmented and occasionally curlier.

The most frequent offenders are chemotherapeutic (anti-cancer) agents and anticoagulants (compounds that prevent or slow the process of blood clotting), but hair loss can occur with a variety of common drugs, a list of which is below.

Some of the myriad medications that can cause hair loss include the following:

## Trade/Brand-names

| | | |
|---|---|---|
| Abilify | Clinoril | Felbatol |
| Accupril | Clomid | Femara |
| Accutane | Colazal | Fludara |
| Aciphex | ColBenemid | Fragmin |
| Actigall | Comvax | FUDR |
| Adriamycin | Concerta | Fungizone |
| Advil | Cordarone | Gabitril |
| Albenza | Coreg | Gemzar |
| Aldara | Cosmegen | Geodon |
| Aleve | Cosopt | Gleevec |
| Alkeran | Coumadin | Gold |
| Altace | Cozaar | Haldol |
| Anaprox | Crixivan | Havrix |
| Androgel | Cymbalta | HCTZ |
| Aralen | Cytosar | Hexalen |
| Arava | Cytotec | Hycamtin |
| Arimidex | Cytovene | Hydrea |
| Aromasin | Cytoxan | Idamycin |
| Asacol | D.T.I.C. | Ifex |
| Azilect | Dacogen | Imuran |
| Azopt | Daypro | Inderal |
| Azulfidine | Decadron | Inhibase |
| Benicar | Depakene | Intron |
| Betagan | Depakote | Invirase |
| Betapace | Desyrel | Keppra |
| BiCNU | Didronel | Kerlone |
| Blenoxane | Diflucan | Kwell |
| Brevibloc | Diovan | Lamictal |
| Capoten | Dipentum | Lamisil |
| Cardizem | Duragesic | Lanoxin |
| Cardura | Elavil | Lariam |
| Casodex | Ellence | Lescol |
| Catapres | Enbrel | Lexapro |
| CeeNU | Epivir | Lipitor |
| Celebrex | Erbitux | Liquemin |
| CellCept | Eskalith | Lithobid |
| Cerubidine | Exovac | Lodine |
| Claritin | Fareston | Loniten |

## Trade/Brand-names

| | | |
|---|---|---|
| Lopid | Parlodel | Sinequan |
| Lopressor | Parnate | Solodyn |
| Lotensin | Peg-Intron | Sonata |
| Lotronex | Pepcid | Soriatane |
| Loxitane | Persantine | Sporanox |
| Lunesta | Pertofrane | SPRYCEL |
| Lupron | Plaquenil | Sular |
| Macrobid | Platinol | Sutent |
| Matulane | Prandin | Synthroid |
| Maxair | Pravachol | Tagamet |
| Mevacor | Prevacid | Tambocor |
| Mexitil | Prexige | Tapazole |
| Miacalcin | Prezista | Tarceva |
| Midamor | Prilosec | Targretin |
| Minipress | Progesterone | Tasmar |
| Minocin | Prograf | Taxol |
| Mitomycin | Propylthiouracil | Taxotere |
| Mobic | Protonix | Tegretol |
| Motrin | Protopic | Temodar |
| Mustargen | Provera | Tenex |
| Myleran | Prozac | Tenormin |
| Nalfon | Purinethol | Tenuate |
| Namenda | Relafen | Teslac |
| Navelbine | Remeron | Testosterone |
| Nexavar | Reyataz | Thioplex |
| Nexium | Rheumatrex | Thyroid |
| Nipent | Rhinocort | Timoptic |
| Nolvadex | Rilutek | Tofranil |
| Normozide | Ritalin | Tonocard |
| Norvasc | Rogaine | Topamax |
| Novantrone | Rythmol | Toprol |
| Omega-3-acids | Salagen | Toradol |
| ethyl esters | Sandostatin | Trecator |
| Orfadin | Sarafem | Tricor |
| Ornidyl | Sectral | Trizivir |
| Orudis | Selenium | Univasc |
| Pamelor | Serzone | Urocid |
| Paraplatin | Sinemet | Valtrex |

## Trade/Brand-names

| | | |
|---|---|---|
| Vasotec | Vitamin B$_3$ | Zestril |
| Velban | Vivactil | Ziac |
| VePesid | Voltaren | Zocor |
| Vermox | Vumon | Zoladex |
| Vfend | Wellbutrin | Zolinza |
| Videx | Xeloda | Zometa |
| Vincasar | Xolair | Zonegran |
| Virazole | Xyrem | Zovirax |
| Visken | Zantac | Zyban |
| Vistide | Zelnorm | Zyrtec |

## Excess Hair

### (Hirsutism; Hypertrichosis)

One of the unhappiest women I know is a young lady with an excess amount of dark hair on her upper lip, her chin, and her chest. She is not alone. There are thousands of young women with the same cosmetic problem: superfluous hair—hair that doesn't look sporty in the locker room; hair where nobody wants it.

Exactly what do we mean by excess hair? Not what most people believe. Excess hair does *not* mean an increase in the number of hairs. Everyone is born with a fixed number of hairs on his or her body. This is genetically determined (inherited).

There are two types of excess hair: one, *hirsutism*, is the growth of excess hair in the areas of the skin, such as the face and chest that are reserved for male hair growth. *Hypertrichosis*, on the other hand, is a disorder where unwanted hair is more or less generalized in distribution. (Hypertrichosis, by the way, also occurs in men.)

Hair grows on every portion of the skin except the palms and soles and a few other small areas. Most of these hairs are of the "peach-fuzz" variety (*vellus* hairs). Others are of the terminal variety—the long, thicker hairs of the scalp (Lady Godiva and Rapunzel), the chest (mostly men), and the pubic region.

Excess hairiness results from the vellus hairs becoming longer, darker, and thicker in areas where one expects to have only peach fuzz.

While excess hair may be due to many factors, for some groups of people it is the normal state of affairs. People from Southern Europe and Middle Eastern cultures are much hairier than those from Northern Europe and Scandinavian countries; white people are hairier than black people; and Asians and Native Americans are the least hairy of all.

Above and beyond this normal, constitutional hairy excess, there are those women who exhibit a far greater increase in the length and thickness of hair in certain areas that are usually reserved for the "peach fuzz" variety: the upper lip, the chin, the sides of the face, the areas around the nipples, and the portion of the abdomen extending from the pubic region to the belly button. (These are the areas normally associated with the male pattern hair growth.) This type of superfluous hair—hirsutism—can be especially embarrassing to the young and otherwise confident woman.

The causes of excess hair are many and varied. For those with a moderate degree of hairiness, the factors involved may be merely a part of normal growth and development. The most common cause of excess hair growth in females is the aging process. During the time of menopause, women become deficient in the production of the female hormone estrogen. The decrease of this hormone gives rise to a relative increase in the male-type hormone (androgen) that is responsible both for the slow, relentless proliferation of thick, dark hairs appearing on the upper lip, chin, and cheeks, and, at the same time, for the beginning of the steady thinning of the scalp hair. These two processes seem to go hand in hand: more hair on the body, less on the scalp.

Stress and tension can also play a role in excess hair growth. The hair follicles are under the influence of various hormones and chemicals produced by the body. Emotional stress and tension often lead to a disturbance in the delicate balance of these hormones which, in turn, can result in a stimulation of the hair follicle leading to excess hair—not, however, on the head. These hormonal imbalances also can arise in connection with tumors and cysts of the ovaries, diseases of the adrenal glands, and abnormal functioning and tumors of other hormone-secreting glands, such as the thyroid or pituitary.

The following may be some of the conditions that may increase a woman's normally low level of male hormones:

- Adrenal hyperplasia (abnormal increase in cells)
- Aging
- Cushing syndrome
- Genetics
- Hormone imbalance
- Insulin resistance
- Medications (see below)
- Obesity
- Polycystic ovary syndrome
- Pregnancy
- Tumors in the ovaries or adrenal gland (cancer)

In addition, various drugs and medications can occasionally produce hypertrichosis when taken over a period of time. These include drugs for epilepsy (Dilantin), cortisone-like drugs, and a host of others..

Some of the medications that have been reported to cause excess hair growth include the following:

### Trade/Brand-names

| Clomid | Neoral | Timoptic |
|---|---|---|
| Cortisone drugs | Rogaine | Topamax |
| Dilantin | Sandimmune | Zyrtec |
| Erbitux | Simulect | |
| Loniten | Soriatane | |

(Note: Many medications have been found to promote long eyelashes. See list under Eyelash Growth in the next section.)

## Eyelash Growth

(Trichomegaly)

Eyelashes—or, simply, lashes—are the rows of the short hairs along the edge of the eyelid that provide natural protection for the eyes from wind, dust, sun, sweat, foreign bodies, insects, and other debris. Lashes perform some of the same function as whiskers do on a cat or a mouse in the sense that they are sensitive to being touched, thus providing a warning that an object (such as an insect or dust mite) is near the eye.

Eyelashes live an average of five or six months, naturally shed about every four to eight weeks, and regrow continually. They have a very short active growth phase, similar to hairs of the arms, legs, and eyebrows, which explains why they are so much shorter than scalp hair.

Abnormally long eyelashes, called *trichomegaly*, are occasionally hereditary, and are sometimes associated with dwarfism. It has reportedly been found in several disorders such as dermatomyositis, uveitis, lupus erythematosus, AIDS, malnutrition, hypothyroidism, and breast cancer, among others. It is also seen during pregnancy. In many cases, this condition runs in families. A new study has revealed that eyelashes of allergic patients were found to be significantly longer than those of non-allergic control subjects.

In an eye disease called *vernal keratoconjunctivitis*, a chronic conjunctivitis that affects children mainly in Mediterranean and other temperate climates, the upper eyelashes are significantly longer than in healthy matched subjects.

Topical latanoprost (Xalatan), a popular intraocular pressure-lowering ophthalmic drug (eye drop) for use in patients with glaucoma and ocular hypertension, has been shown to increase number, length, thickness, curvature, and pigmentation of eyelashes. This lengthening is occasionally persistent even after the medication is discontinued. The new growth of lashlike hair may include extra rows of eyelashes. Bimatoprost (Lumigan), another eyedrop, can cause increased hair growth of the eyelashes as well as over the upper cheek region. Travoprost (Travatan) eyedrops have also been reported to cause eyelash growth.

Drugs that have been reported to cause excess lengthening of eyelashes include the following:

## Trade/Brand-names

| | | |
|---|---|---|
| Clomid | Loniten | Soriatane |
| Cosopt | Lumigan | Timoptic |
| Cortisone-like | Neoral | Topamax |
|    drugs | Rogaine | Trusopt |
| Dilantin | Sandimmune | Xalatan |
| Erbitux | Simulect | Zyrtec |

# PART C
## MOUTH/TONGUE/
## TEETH/GUM
## DISORDERS

# Chapter 1:  Mouth

## Burning Mouth/Tongue Syndrome (BMS)

(Stomatopyrosis; Stomatodynia; Glossopyrosis;
Glossodynia)

Burning mouth/tongue syndrome (BMS) is a complex, disturbing malady in which a burning pain occurs that may, in the absence of any specific oral lesions, involve the tongue, lips, or the whole mouth. Synonyms for BMS are stomatopyrosis (literally means "burning mouth"), stomatodynia ("painful mouth"), glossopyrosis ("burning tongue"), and glossodynia ("painful tongue"). These terms are often used interchangeably by many physicians and dentists. Other names occasionally used under the BMS rubric include scalded mouth syndrome and burning lips syndrome.

The precise cause of this commonly misdiagnosed, overlooked, and often poorly managed condition is difficult to ascertain. It is especially common in women after menopause. Many patients show depression associated with anxiety, with evidence of psychiatric disorders in the family. In the geriatric population, it often persists for months or years.

BMS is typically characterized by an unremitting and often intense burning sensation of the mouth or tongue as if it was scalded or on fire. Acidic foods such as tomatoes, orange juice, and lemons cause considerable distress. In some, the pain is almost nonexistent in the morning but builds up over the course of the day; in others the pain is uninterrupted throughout the day. Other symptoms can include dry mouth (xerostomia), a numb or tingling sensation in the mouth or on the tip of the tongue, and a metallic or bitter taste.

The prevalence of BMS reported in some recent studies ranges between 1 and 5 percent of the general population and is uncommon before the age of thirty. The onset in women usually occurs within three to twelve years after menopause. It has been reported in 10 to 40 percent of women seeking treatment for menopausal symptoms. More than one million American adults are afflicted with this unpleasant and incapacitating disorder.

The most frequent associated conditions of burning pain include the following:
- Aging
- Allergies or reactions to food
- Amalgam fillings
- Anxiety, depression, or other emotional disorders
- Bruxism (grinding teeth) (q.v.)
- Candidiasis (yeast infection)
- Diabetes and/or diabetic neuropathy
- Excessive irritation from extreme brushing of tongue

- Gastro-esophageal reflux disease—GERD (acid reflux)
- Geographic tongue
- Hormonal changes associated with menopause
- Hypersensitivity reactions
- Local oral infections by yeast (thrush)
- Medications (see below)
- Menopause
- Mercury allergy
- Nerve damage of the tongue
- Nickel allergy
- Nutritional deficiencies (Vitamin B complex; iron; zinc)
- Overuse of mouthwashes
- Peanut sensitivity
- Poor-fitting or irritating dentures
- Psychogenic disorders (depression, anxiety, fear of cancer)
- Psychosocial stresses (stressful life events such as bereavement)
- Sjøgren's syndrome
- Xerostomia (dry mouth), often related to medications

BMS is a major diagnostic problem. Treatment is still unsatisfactory and there is no definitive cure. In the short term, people may gain some relief by avoiding irritating substances such as alcohol-based mouthwashes, cinnamon or mint products, and cigarette smoke. Chewing on ice chips or sugar-free gum, keeping dentures out all night, and brushing the teeth with baking soda might also help.

Medications that have been reported to bring about burning mouth/tongue syndrome include the following:

## Trade/Brand-names

| | | |
|---|---|---|
| ACE-inhibitors | Mercury | Sustiva |
| Atacand | Neurontin | Teveten |
| Cephalosporins | Pamelor | Vasotec |
| Chloroptic | Penicillin | Viramune |
| Gold | Prinivil | Zephrex |
| Klonopin | Sinequan | Zestril |

## Black Hairy Tongue

(Lingua Villosa Nigra)

Black hairy tongue—also called "black tongue"—refers to a number of conditions that cause the tongue to become unusually dark and/or hairy in appearance. This coating is usually located in the middle to the back of the tongue. While brownish black is the most common color associated with this disorder, other colors—brown, white, yellow, green, or pink have also been recorded.

A black, hairy tongue customarily results from an excess growth of bacteria, and sometimes yeasts, that typically live in the mouth. It is a short-lived, harmless, asymptomatic condition. These organisms collect on the surface of the tongue, which has hundreds of tiny fingerlike projections, *filiform papillae*, and cause a change of color. Certain types of bacteria and yeasts make blood cell pigments that can give the tongue a black appearance. In some cases, the tongue may also seem "hairy" due to more rapid growth of papillae or a disruption of the normal shedding of cells by the tongue. The top layers normally wear away, but in some instances these cells are not sloughed off and the papillae grow longer. These papillae then trap bacteria and other organisms giving the tongue a furry or hairy impression—like moss developing on a rock. The black color is a result of the color of the bacteria which appear dark or black. Secondary infections with yeastlike organisms—

*Candida albicans*—can supervene. This condition is commonly known as *thrush*.

In some cases, the origin of the black, coated tongue can not be determined. However, some potential causes include the following:
- Changes in the normal bacteria or yeast population of the mouth following antibiotic treatment
- Chronic use of oral antibiotics
- Dehydration
- Drinking excessive amounts of coffee or tea
- Dry mouth
- Medications containing bismuth, such as Pepto-Bismol
- Aging
- Poor oral hygiene
- Radiation therapy to the head or neck
- Regular use of mouthwashes containing peroxide, witch hazel, or menthol
- Tobacco smokers
- Uncontrolled diabetes

Bad breath *(halitosis)* and distorted taste *(dysgeusia)* are the only symptoms associated with black hairy tongue; both of these symptoms are discussed elsewhere in this book.

The occurrence of black hairy tongue varies widely, from about 8 percent in children and young adults to 57 percent in persons who are addicted to drugs. Hairy tongue has been reported with greater frequency in males.

Medications reported to cause black hairy tongue include the following:

## Trade/Brand-names

| | | |
|---|---|---|
| Amoxil | Pamelor | Sinemet |
| Augmentin | PEG-Intron | Surmontil |
| Avelox | Penicillin | Thelin |
| Biaxin | Pepto-Bismol | Tindamax |
| Dyazide | Pertofrane | Tofranil |
| Dyrenium | Prevacid | Vistide |
| Elavil | Protonix | Zithromax |
| Exovac | Prozac | Zyprexa |
| Kepivance | Remeron | Zyrtec |
| Marplan | Risperdal | Zyvox |
| Maxzide | Rocephin | |
| Minocin | Sarafem | |

## Canker Sores

(Aphthous Stomatitis)

> Roses have thorns, and silver fountains
>     of mud;
> Clouds and eclipses stain both moon and
>     sun,
> And loathsome canker lives in sweetest
>     bud.
> All men make faults.
> —William Shakespeare, Sonnet 35

Canker sores are painful ulcerations in the mouth affecting about 25 percent of the population. Even the ancient Greeks were plagued by mouth ulcers. The medical term for this baffling condition, coined by Hippocrates in the fourth century BCE, is *aphthous stomatitis*—but these sores by any other name are just as painful.

Many people confuse canker sores with cold sores. They are not the same. A virus causes cold sores. But we know little about what causes canker sores and even less about what cures them. Nor do we know what prevents them. We *do* know that they are not contagious, they are more common in women, they are not hereditary, and they do *not* cause cancer.

Canker sores develop as small blisters in the mouth, singly or in groups, which usually go unnoticed. These blisters break and small, round, shallow ulcers develop. The ulcers gradually enlarge and become yellow and shiny with bright red borders. They can be exquisitely tender and painful—so painful sometimes that it can severely disrupt a person's eating.

Canker sores can be found anywhere in the mouth: the inside of the cheeks, the lips, the sides of the tongue, the floor of the mouth, the gums, and the palate. They heal by themselves in about two weeks without leaving scars. Unfortunately, however, they tend to recur. Some people develop them every few weeks, others every few months, and some unlucky few are never without them.

Although no one knows what causes these painful mouth sores, many of the following triggering factors have been suspected:

- Allergies to drugs, such as aspirin, antibiotics, sulfa drugs, and chemotherapeutic agents to treat cancer (see list on page 172)
- Bacteria
- Fatigue, emotional stress, and tension
- Foods such as chocolate, citrus fruits, spices, milk, cola drinks, and nuts, especially English walnuts
- Febrile illnesses
- Injury caused by stiff toothbrushes, poorly fitting dentures, as well as certain denture materials
- Menstruation
- Poor dental hygiene and inadequate or improper brushing and flossing
- Viruses (similar to the viral infection responsible for cold sores)

Many patients have told me—and other doctors—that shortly after they had given up smoking, they began to develop canker sores. And when they started to smoke again, the sores disappeared never to return. (However, I do not recommend smoking to alleviate or prevent canker sores based on these apocryphal and scientifically untested accounts!)

Medications that have been reported to trigger canker sores include the following:

### Trade/Brand-names

| | | |
|---|---|---|
| Advil | Gold | Protonix |
| Aldara | Habitrol | Prozac |
| Aleve | Hepatitis B vaccine | Rapamune |
| Ansaid | Hivid | Remeron |
| Aspirin | Hyzaar | Rescriptor |
| Astelin | Imuran | Reyataz |
| Atacand | Indocin | Rheumatrex |
| Azactam | Intron A | Sarafem |
| Azulfidine | Lamisil | Septra |
| Bactrin | Licorice | Seromycin |
| Benzocaine | Lyrica | Sinequan |
| Capoten | Meclofenamate | Syprine |
| Clinoril | Motrin | Tarceva |
| Co-trimoxazole | Mycobutin | Taxotere |
| Cozaar | Nalfon | Thalidomide |
| Crixivan | Naprosyn | Tolectin |
| Cymbalta | Nicoderm | Toradol |
| Depen | Nicoran | Tysabri |
| Diovan | Orudis | Varicella vaccine |
| Dolobid | Paxil | Vioxx |
| Echinacea | Pediazole | Vistide |
| Erbitux | PEG-intron | Voltaren |
| Feldene | Prograf | Zoloft |
| Fluorides | Proleukin | Zyprexa |

## Drooling

### (Sialorrhea, Hypersalivation, Ptyalism)

Drooling (also known as sialorrhea, hypersalivation, and ptyalism) occurs when saliva dribbles outside the margin of the lower lip. Drooling is usually caused by excessive production of saliva, inability to keep saliva within the mouth, or difficulties with swallowing. Drooling is a significant problem in children who are afflicted with mental retardation or cerebral palsy as well as in adults who have Parkinsonism or have had a stroke.

The function of saliva, the watery and usually frothy substance produced in the mouth, is to lubricate and moisten food in order to assist in mastication. Saliva also has bacteriostatic and bactericidal properties that are important for maintaining oral health and function and that helps lessen mouth odor.

While drooling is a normal occurrence in children before the age of twenty-four months, drooling after age four is uniformly considered abnormal. Drooling causes functional, social, psychological, and clinical responsibilities on patients, their families, and caregivers.

Patients often succumb to recurrent skin breakdown; their cheeks become dry and chapped; secondary infection often supervenes; foul odors develop; and clothing and bibs become soiled and require frequent changing. Social embarrassment makes it challenging for patients to interact with their peers; this can lead to seclusion. Caretakers and family may find it more difficult to show affection with these patients, contributing to a potentially destructive stigmatization.

Disorders associated with drooling include the following:
- Cerebral palsy
- Dental malocclusion or other orthodontic problems
- Gastroesophageal reflux (GERD)
- Head and neck surgical defects ("Andy Gump" deformity)
- Medication side effects (see top of page 174)

- Mental retardation
- Parkinsonism
- Pregnancy
- Stroke
- Toxin exposure (mercury vapor)

Drugs that have been reported to induce drooling to a clinically significant degree include the following:

### Trade/Brand-names

| | | |
|---|---|---|
| Capoten | Lithobid | Urecholine |
| Catapres | Luvox | Urised |
| Clozaril | Mercury | Yohimbine |
| Eskalith | Risperdal | Zyprexa |
| Haldol | Sinemet | |

## Dry Mouth

(Xerostomia)

Dry mouth—*xerostomia*—is defined as a lack of saliva flow. It is the condition of not having enough saliva—spit—to keep the mouth wet. Xerostomia is sometimes colloquially called "pasties," "cottonmouth," or "doughmouth."

Dry mouth can cause difficulty in chewing, eating, swallowing, and talking. It also leads to halitosis (bad breath) and increases the risk for tooth decay because saliva helps keep in check the harmful germs that cause cavities. It is a common complaint found often among older adults, affecting approximately 20 percent of the elderly. This may be the result of polypharmacy (the practice of taking too many medications).

Although xerostomia may be a sign of an underlying disease, such as Sjøgren's syndrome, anemia, cystic fibrosis, rheumatoid arthritis, and poorly controlled diabetes, common habits such as tobacco smoking, alcohol use (including those in mouthwashes), excessive mouth breathing, dehydration, and the consumption of beverages containing caffeine can cause oral dryness. The most common cause of reduced salivation, however, is medication. In the elderly using over-the-counter products—most frequently, dimenhydrinate (21 percent), acetaminophen (paracetamol) (19 percent), diphenhydramine (15 percent), alcohol (13 percent), and herbal products (11 percent)—dry mouth is very common. A symptom of methamphetamine abuse usually called "meth mouth" is largely caused by xerostomia.

Xerostomia often occurs along with other symptoms:
- Bad breath
- Burning or tingling sensation, especially on the tongue
- Difficulty in swallowing
- Difficulty wearing dentures
- Dry nasal passages
- Dry, cracked lips
- Frequent thirst
- Increase in dental problems, such as cavities and periodontal disease
- Red, raw tongue
- Repeated yeast infections in the mouth
- Sore throat and hoarseness
- Sores in mouth or at corners of lips
- Speech problems
- Taste problems

Hundreds of drugs can cause dry mouth. The *categories* of medications responsible for dry mouth include the following:
- ACE-inhibitors
- Antidepressants
- Antihistamines
- Anti-HIV drugs
- Antihypertensives
- Antimigraine drugs
- Antipsychotics

- Appetite suppressants
- Bronchodilators
- Cytotoxic drugs
- Decongestants and "cold cures"
- Diuretics
- H2 receptor antagonists and proton-pump inhibitors
- Medications used to treat overactive bladder
- Opioids, benzodiazepines, hypnotics, and drugs of abuse
- Retinoids (a class of chemicals related to Vitamin A)
- Skeletal muscle relaxants

The list of *specific* medications responsible for dry mouth is as follows:

### Trade/Brand-names

| | | |
|---|---|---|
| Abilify | Antivert | BuSpar |
| Accupril | Arava | Campral |
| Accutane | Arimidex | Cantil |
| Aceon | Asacol | Capoten |
| Actifed | Astelin | Carafate |
| Adderall | Atarax | Cardene |
| Adipex-P | Ativan | Cardura |
| Adrenaline | Atrovent | Casodex |
| Adriamycin | Avastin | Catapres |
| Aerobid | Axert | Celebrex |
| Akineton | Axid | Celexa |
| Aldomet | Azilect | Cerubidine |
| Aleve | Azopt | Chantix |
| Allegra | Benadryl | Cialis |
| Aloxi | Bentyl | Clarinex |
| Alphagan | Betapace | Claritin |
| Altace | Bismuth | Clozaril |
| Ambien | Bontril | Codeine |
| Amitiza | Botox | Cogentin |
| Amoxapine | Brethine | Colazal |
| Anafranil | Brevibloc | Compazine |

## Trade/Brand-names

| | | |
|---|---|---|
| Coreg | Focalin | Maxair |
| Cosopt | Fuzeon | Maxalt |
| Cozaar | Geodon | Mellaril |
| Cubicin | Halcion | Meridia |
| Cymbalta | Haldol | Mevacor |
| Darvon | HCTZ | Mexitil |
| Daypro | Hytrin | Miacalcin |
| Demerol | Imitrex | Migranal |
| Desoxyn | Insulin | Minipress |
| Desyrel | Intron A | Minocin |
| Detrol | Invega | Mirapex |
| Dimetane | Inversine | Moban |
| Diovan | Isordil | Mobic |
| Dipentum | Ivanz | Monopril |
| Ditropan | Kemadrin | Morphine |
| Dolophine | Ketek | MS Contin |
| Doral | Klonopin | Myleran |
| Dostinex | Lamictal | Nalfon |
| Dramamine | Levatol | Nardil |
| Duragesic | Levitra | Navane |
| Effexor | Levsinex | Neoral |
| Elavil | Lexapro | Neupro |
| Eldepryl | Librax | Nexavar |
| Enablex | Librium | Nexium |
| Enbrel | Lioresal | Nicoderm |
| Erbitux | Lipitor | Nicotine |
| Ethyol | Lithium | Nitrostat |
| Evoxin | Lithobid | Norflex |
| Exovac | Lomotil | Noroxin |
| Fansidar | Loxitane | Norpace |
| Felbatol | Lozol | Norvasc |
| Femara | Ludiomil | Norvir |
| Fiorinal | Lunesta | Novahistine |
| Flagyl | Luvox | Noxafil |
| Flexeril | Lyrica | Nubain |
| Flomax | Marinol | Nuvigil |
| Floxin | Marplan | Omnicef |
| Flumadine | Matulane | Orap |

## Trade/Brand-names

| | | |
|---|---|---|
| Orudis | Robinul | Tofranil |
| Oxeze | Romazicon | Tonocard |
| OxyContin | Rondec | Topamax |
| Pamelor | Rynatuss | Toprol |
| Pardolel | Rythmol | Toradol |
| Parnate | Salagen | Trans-Scop |
| Paxil | Sandostatin | Transtex |
| PEG-Intron | Sectral | Tranxene |
| Pepcid | Serax | Trental |
| Periactin | Serevent | Trihexy |
| Permax | Seroquel | Trilafon |
| Pertofrane | Serpasil | Trisonex |
| Phenergan | Serzone | Tylenol |
| Polaramine | Sinemet | Ultram |
| Prezista | Sinequan | Urispas |
| Prialt | Skelid | Valium |
| Prilosec | Sonata | Vascase |
| Proamatine | Soriatane | Vasotec |
| Progesterone | Spiriva | Vesicare |
| Prolixin | Stelazine | Vfend |
| Propantheline | Strattera | Vicodin |
| ProSom | Sudafed | Videx |
| Protonix | Sular | Virazole |
| Proventil | Surmontil | Vivactil |
| Provigil | Sutent | Voltaren |
| Prozac | Symmetrel | Vyvanse |
| Ranexa | Talwin | Wellbutrin |
| Reglan | Tambocor | Xanax |
| Relafen | Tarceva | Xopenex |
| Relpax | Targretin | Xyzal |
| Remeron | Tasmar | Zaditor |
| Reminyl | Tavist | Zanaflex |
| ReoPro | Tegretol | Zaroxolyn |
| Requip | Tenex | Zestril |
| Restoril | Tenuate | Ziac |
| Revlimid | Thlidomid | Zofran |
| Rexitene | Thorazine | Zoladex |
| Risperdal | Timoptic | Zolinza |

Trade/Brand-names

| | | |
|---|---|---|
| Zoloft | Zonegran | Zyrtec |
| Zometa | Zyban | |
| Zomig | Zyprexa | |

## Halitosis

### (Bad Breath, Foetor Oris, Foetor Ex Ore)

Halitosis, bad breath, foetor ex ore, and foetor oris are terms—among others—that are used to describe noticeably unpleasant odors exhaled in breathing—stale or foul-smelling breath—whether the smell is or is not from an oral source. Bad breath may be a sign of a health problem.

About 90 percent of bad breath originates in the mouth. Food sticks between your teeth, around the gums, and on your tongue. If you don't brush and floss your teeth at least every day, this food breaks down and rots causing bad breath.

Chronic bad breath affects about 25 percent of the population in varying degrees. It can negatively affect the individual's personal, social, and business relationships, and can lead to poor self-esteem and increased stress. Halitosis has a significant impact on those who suffer from it or believe they do (halitophobia) and is estimated to be the third most frequent reason for seeking dental advice.

What you eat and drink affects your breath. Once food is digested and its oils are absorbed into the bloodstream, they're carried into the lungs and the odor is given off in your breath.

Bad breath may be caused by the following:
- A foreign object lodged in the nose, such as a bean
- Bronchitis and other upper respiratory infections
- Cancers
- Canker sores
- Chronic lung infections and lung abscesses

- Crash dieting (Dieters may develop unpleasant "fruity" breath from ketoacidosis, the breakdown of chemicals during fasting.)
- Dental problems: poor dental hygiene and periodontal disease (Without brushing and flossing daily, food particles remain in their mouth and a colorless, sticky film of bacteria (plaque) forms on the teeth. If not brushed away, plaque can irritate the gums (gingivitis) and cause tooth decay. Plaque-filled pockets can form between the teeth and gums (periodontitis), worsening this problem—and the breath. Dentures that aren't cleaned regularly or don't fit correctly also can hide odor-causing bacteria and food particles.)
- Diabetes
- Dry mouth (Saliva helps cleanse and moisten the mouth. A dry mouth allows dead cells to accumulate on the tongue, gums, and cheeks. These cells then decompose; this causes odor. Dry mouth, the reason for "morning breath" also known as "Dragon Breath," occurs during sleep.)
- Excessive bacterial growth on the back of the tongue
- Food: particularly onions, garlic, fish, and cheeses (After these foods are digested and the oils absorbed into the bloodstream, they are transported to the lungs and are released in the breath until the food is eliminated from the body. Alcohol is absorbed in the same way, allowing the measurement of alcohol levels by breathalyzer tests.)
- Hiatal hernia
- Kidney infections and failure (can cause a urinelike odor), and liver failure (which may cause an odor described as "fishy.")
- Medications (see list on page 182)
- Mononucleosis

- Mouth, nose, and throat disorders
- Periodontal disease
- Acid reflux (GERD)
- Respiratory tract infections
- Sinus infections
- Strep throat
- Tobacco products (Smoking dries out the mouth and causes its own unpleasant mouth odor. Tobacco users are also more likely to have periodontal disease, itself a cause of bad breath.)
- Tongue coating
- Tonsillitis
- *Trimethylaminuria* ("fish odor syndrome")

Bad breath has been with us since the beginning of time. The problem is discussed at length in the Jewish Talmud as well as by Greek and Roman writers. Islam emphasizes fresh breath in the context of good oral hygiene. The prophet Mohammed is said to have thrown a churchgoer from the roof of a mosque for having the smell of garlic on his breath. The activity of keeping the mouth clean and fresh dates all the way back to Gautama Buddha (in the fifth or sixth century BCE) who would use a "tooth stick" from the God Sakka as part of his personal hygiene regimen.

Ancient folk remedies, many of which are stll in use, are plentiful. The book of Genesis mentions labdanum (mastic), a resin derived from the *Pistacia lentiscus* tree, which has been used in Mediterranean countries for breath freshening for thousands of years. Other folk cures include parsley (Italy), cloves (Iraq), guava peels (Thailand), and eggshells (China). Ancient medical writers such as the Greek physician Hippocrates and the Roman physician Pliny (23–70 CE) wrote about cures for sweetening the breath. As early as 2,000 to 3,000 years ago writers wrote about natural remedies such as peppermint for bad breath.

The Listerine saga: Listerine was originally invented in the nineteenth century as a powerful surgical antiseptic. It was later sold from time to time as a floor cleaner and subsequently as a cure for gonorrhea. But it wasn't a success until the 1920s, when it was promoted as the universal cure for "chronic halitosis." The makers of Listerine launched an ad campaign in 1921 that played heavily on the angst about how others would react to a halitosis victim. The most famous of their ads, for their Listerine mouthwash, concerned the pathetic case of "Edna, who was often a bridesmaid but never a bride." She was closing in on her "tragic" thirtieth birthday unmarried because she suffered from halitosis—a disorder that "you, yourself, rarely know when you have it. And even your closest friends won't tell you."

Some celebrities are rumored to have been afflicted with halitosis, including Hugh Grant, Ben Affleck, and the late Clark Gable. In October, 1999, Larry King had been interviewing Donald Trump. Though King usually asked the questions, Trump had an awkward question of his own. "Do you mind if I sit back a little?" he asked, and then added, "Because your breath is very bad."

Medications that have been reported to cause halitosis include the following:

### Trade/Brand-names

| | | |
|---|---|---|
| Azactam | Imovane | Protonix |
| DMSO | Lamictal | Selenium |
| Garlic | Prevacid | Serzone |

# Chapter 2: Teeth and Gums

## Clenching and Grinding Teeth

(Bruxism)

> But the children of the kingdom shall be
> cast out into the outer darkness: There
> shall be weeping and gnashing of teeth.
> —Matthew 8:12

*Bruxism* is the technical term for an involuntary gnashing, grinding, or clenching of teeth. It is more often than not an unconscious activity, whether the person is awake or asleep. Frequently associated with fatigue, anxiety, pain, stress, or fear, it often causes malocclusion of the teeth. This usually results in abnormal wear-patterns on the teeth, periodontal breakdown, or mandibular joint problems.

Between 20 and 50 percent of people with bruxism have at least one close relative with a history of grinding teeth. Bruxism affects nearly all Down syndrome children and adults. Many skulls of cavemen exhibit short, flat teeth and some primitive cave dwellers ground their teeth away altogether probably in a combination with a harsh diet and poor dental hygiene.

Mona Lisa is said to have been a "bruxer." The "grind" of posing may have led to Mona Lisa's somewhat odd smile. An Italian doctor, Filippo Surano, believes that the noblewoman in Leonardo da Vinci's portrait suffered from bruxism. Surano says the strain of posing for the painting could have triggered an attack of teeth grinding.

There are seven passages in the New Testament that speak of "weeping and gnashing of teeth." Six are found in the gospel of Matthew, one in Luke.

Bruxism (from the Greek, *brugmós*, a gnashing) is typically accompanied by clenching of the jaw. It is one of the oldest ailments known, and approximately one in four adults experiences it. Bruxism occurs an average of twenty-five times per night, in four to five-second episodes. Thus, people with bruxism may grind their teeth for more than two minutes during just one night's sleep. Even during short naps, most people are not conscious of grinding their teeth until they have been noticeably damaged. This unconscious behavior is perhaps a release of aggression, angst, or anger. Bruxism is a common sleep disorder: thirty to forty million Americans grind their teeth during sleep.

In most people, bruxism is mild enough not to be a health problem; however, some people suffer from significant bruxism that can become symptomatic. Symptoms such as moderate to severe headache, muscle pain, temporomandibular joint dysfunction, and permanent tooth and jaw damage may supervene if bruxism is left untreated.

Those medications that have been implicated in inducing bruxism include the following:

## Trade/Brand-names

| | | |
|---|---|---|
| Celexa | Effexor | Ritalin |
| Concerta | Eldepryl | Sarafem |
| Cymbalta | Haldol | Wellbutrin |
| Depakene | Lexapro | Zoloft |
| Depakote | Luvox | Zyban |
| Desoxyn | Paxil | |
| Ecstacy | Prozac | |

## Tooth Pigmentation

(Colored Teeth)

Tooth discoloration can be caused by many different factors. Some influence the formation of the enamel, while others cause the staining of enamel. Discoloration may be uniform or may appear as spots or lines in the enamel. Discolored areas may also have a different density and porosity than normal enamel.

Factors determining tooth color include genetic, congenital (existing at birth), infectious, and environmental. Inherited diseases may influence the thickness of enamel or the calcium or protein content of the enamel. Metabolic diseases (diseases caused by malfunctions in body processes), may cause both abnormalities of color and shape.

Drugs and medications either taken by the mother while pregnant or by the child during the time of tooth development can cause changes in both the color and hardness of the enamel (see list provided on page 186).

The following medical conditions may cause tooth discoloration:

- Aging
- Calcium metabolism disorders
- Certain foods
- Certain medications (see list on page 186)
- Chewing tobacco
- Chlorhexidine mouth rinsing
- Dead tooth (the tooth looks gray)
- Excessive coffee and tea drinking
- Fluoride treatment (applications, rinses, toothpastes, supplements)
- Fungal infection
- Injured tooth
- Maternal tetracyclines during pregnancy
- Mercury dental amalgam
- Poor oral and dental hygiene

- *Porphyria,* a disease characterized by an excessive production of pigmentation in the body
- Rickets
- Smoking
- Tetracycline administration in children under age eight
- Tooth abscess

Intrinsic discoloration occurs following a change to the structural composition or thickness of the dental hard tissues. The normal color of teeth is determined by the blue, green, and pink tints of the enamel and is reinforced by the yellow through to brown shades of dentine beneath (dentine is the hard, bony material beneath the enamel of a tooth). A number of metabolic diseases and systemic factors are known to affect the developing dentition and cause discoloration as a consequence. Local factors such as injury are also recognized.

Medications that have been reported to cause tooth staining include the following:

### Trade/Brand-names

| | | |
|---|---|---|
| Accupril | Didronel | Pentam-300 |
| Aceon | Lamisil | Primaxin |
| Altace | Lunesta | Rythmol |
| Amoxil | Minocin | Tarka |
| Biaxin | Monodox | Vasotec |
| Cipro | Monopril | Zestril |
| Declomycin | Orfadin | |

## Swollen Gums

(Gingival Enlargement; Gingival Hyperplasia)

Swollen gums, technically called either *gingival enlargement*, *gingival hyperplasia*, or *gingival hypertrophy*, was first described in the dental literature in the early 1960s in epileptic children receiving therapy with phenytoin (Dilantin) for the management of epilepsy (convulsions). Gingival enlargement is excessive overgrowth of the gum tissue—the *gingiva*—which are part of the soft tissue lining of the mouth that surround the teeth and provide a seal around them. Half of all people who take phenytoin will develop gingival enlargement. Other medications have since been reported to trigger a similar reaction (see list on page 188).

In gingival enlargement, the gingiva can often completely cover the teeth. This growth is usually irregular and may or may not be associated with bleeding.

Gingival enlargement has often been associated with any of the following:

- Blood dyscrasias (abnormal conditions of the blood)
- Benign tumors, such as fibromas, papillomas, and granulomas
- Diabetes (uncontrolled)
- Gingivitis
- Inadequate nutrition
- Leukemias
- Medications (see list on page 188)
- Poor oral hygiene
- Pregnancy
- Puberty
- Sarcoidosis
- Tuberculosis
- Vitamin C deficiency (scurvy)

The list of the medications that can trigger gingival enlargement follows:

## Trade/Brand-names

| | | |
|---|---|---|
| Adalat | Lipitor | Sabril |
| Bactrim | Lithobid | Septra |
| Calan | Lomotil | Simulect |
| Cardene | Lotensin | Sular |
| Cardizem | Milontin | Taxol |
| Celontin | Mysoline | Teczem |
| Depakene | Neoral | Tegretol |
| Depakote | Nizoral | Tiazac |
| Dilantin | Norvasc | Topamax |
| Diovan | Oral contraceptives | Vascor |
| DynaCirc | Orap | Vasotec |
| Erythromycin | Peganone | Zarontin |
| Eskalith | Phenobarbital | Zithromax |
| Exovac | Plendil | Zoloft |
| Felbatol | Prograf | Zonegran |
| Intron A | Rapamune | |
| Lamictal | Rheumatrex | |

# PART D
# HEARING
# DISORDERS

## Hearing Loss

(Deafness)

> Heard melodies are sweet, but those
>   unheard
> Are sweeter; therefore, ye soft pipes, play
>   on . . .
> —John Keats, "Ode on a Grecian Urn"

A hearing impairment or hearing loss is a partial or full decrease in the ability to detect or understand sounds. More than thirty-five million Americans have significant hearing loss. That's more than one in eight individuals. Hearing loss occurs as we age; it is one of the most common conditions affecting older adults. About one-third of Americans between the ages of sixty-five and seventy-four have hearing problems. Among seniors, hearing loss is the third most prevalent complaint, behind arthritis and hypertension. About half of people eighty-five and older have hearing loss.

Hearing loss is not only age-related. It can occur as a result of physical problems with the movement of sound through the ear as occurs with gradual buildup of ear wax that blocks the ear canal or the presence of a foreign body.

Causes of hearing loss include the following:
- Allergies
- Autoimmune diseases

- Bacterial and viral infections
- Benign tumors
- Diabetes
- Excessive noise (power saws, motorcycle riding, rock concerts, boom boxes)
- Genetic disorders
- Head or face trauma
- Leukemia
- Loud explosions
- Pressure trauma (as with sea divers)
- Ruptured eardrum from a middle ear infection
- Sickle-cell anemia
- Simple blows to the head
- Use of cotton swabs
- Various ototoxic—ear-damaging—medications (see list on page 192)

Soldiers and marines caught in roadside bombings and fire-fights in Iraq and Afghanistan have come home in epidemic numbers with permanent hearing loss and ringing in their ears. Hearing damage is their number one disability.

When someone in the family has a hearing loss, the entire family has a hearing problem. An untreated hearing loss is more noticeable than hearing aids.

Celebrities with hearing problems:
- Arnold Palmer
- Dwight D. Eisenhower
- Japanese pop princess Ayumi Hamasaki
- Martin Luther
- Ronald Reagan (In 1983 President Reagan was fitted with hearing aids according to Dr. John House, his ear physician. He had a right ear hearing loss for many years as a result of exposure to gunshot noise while filming westerns.)
- Rush Limbaugh
- Thomas Edison

Throughout history and right up until the 1950s, hearing people believed deafness to be so terrible it had to be "cured" in any way imaginable, even if the cure risked bodily harm. The following are some of the "cures," from quacks, old wives' tales, and superstitions:

- Climb up very, very high then suddenly jump down. The sharp fall will restore the hearing.
- Cut the body and let out some blood (bloodletting). This will cure deafness.
- Electrical treatments have been used to cure deafness. (Called "electromedicine.")
- Fry peach kernels in hog lard and put drops in the ear until deafness is cured.
- Heat your urine using two dishes, and use the water that boils off, in the ear. The water in the ear will stop the deafness.
- Let yourself be hypnotized; when you come out of it, you will hear again.
- Mix your urine with garlic and olive oil and stir gently. Drink this 3 times a day and you will be cured.
- Sit in a chair for three days and three nights without food or water and deafness will be cured.
- Stick a twig in the ear and keep it there all day and night until the deafness is cured.
- Take a certain brand of snuff. It will cure you of deafness.
- Take opium. The drug will cure deafness.
- While yawning put pepper in mouth and the sneeze will take away your deafness.

## Trivia:
- Animals hear more sounds than humans.
- At higher elevations, the change in pressure causes your ears to pop.

- Babies can get earaches because of milk backing up in the eustachian tube, which may cause hearing problems later in life.
- Children have more sensitive ears than adults; they can recognize a wider variety of noises.
- Dolphins have the best sense of hearing among animals; they are able to hear 14 times better than humans.

Medications that have been reported to cause loss of hearing include the following:

### Trade/Brand-names

| | | |
|---|---|---|
| Advil | Floxin | Orudis |
| Aleve | Fludara | PEG-Intron |
| Altace | Fungizone | Pepto-Bismol |
| Amikin | Garamycin | Platinol |
| Ancobon | Imitrex | Ponstel |
| Ansaid | Indocin | Quinora |
| Aralen | Intron-A | Raptiva |
| Aspirin | Kantrex | Relafen |
| Azulfidine | Lasix | Streptomycin |
| Biaxin | Levitra | Taxol |
| Botox | Lodine | Taxotere |
| Cialis | Matulane | Tobradex |
| Clinoril | Meclofenamate | Tolectin |
| Combivir | Miacalcin | Topamax |
| Daypro | Minocin | Toradol |
| Desferal | Motrin | Vancocin |
| Desoxyn | Nalfon | Viagra |
| Dolobid | Naprosyn | Virazole |
| Edecrin | Neoral | Vistide |
| Erythromycin | Neosporin | Visudyne |
| Exjade | Neurontin | Voltaren |
| Feldene | Noroxin | Zithromax |

## Tinnitus

### (Ringing in the Ears)

Tinnitus (from the Latin word "to tinkle or ring like a bell") is the perception of sound—ringing, buzzing, hissing, humming, whistling, whining, roaring, ticking, clicking, banging, beeping, or pulsating—in the human ear, when none exists. It has also been described as a "whooshing" sound, like wind or waves, "crickets" or "tree frogs" or "locusts." To some it's a chirping, clanging, sizzling, rumbling, or a dreadful shrieking noise. The sound perceived may range from a quiet background noise to one that can be heard even over loud extraneous sounds and can be sensed in one or both ears or, rarely, inside the head. And it can be like rushing water, breaking glass, or chain saws running.

Tinnitus is and has probably always been a very common phenomenon. The disorder has affected people since ancient times. Descriptions of tinnitus have been found on Babylonian clay tablets, and the disorder was also known among the Sumerians and in ancient Egypt.

A link between hearing loss and tinnitus was reportedly established for the first time in ancient India in the Ayurveda science. In China, tinnitus was considered a consequence of the disturbed interplay of Yin and Yang. In Greco-Roman antiquity, people affected by tinnitus were ascribed the faculty of hearing divine sounds—"cosmic music" according to Plato and Pythagoras. Hippocrates, in 400 BCE, declared that "Tinnitus is the little brother of epilepsy."

Tinnitus is a malady that affects millions of people all over the world, so its occurrence among the famous comes as no surprise. Many prominent people and celebrities have been and are still tormented by this disorder. Tinnitus is common among musicians.

Some well-known people with tinnitus are:

## Actors, Actresses, Singers, TV and Radio Personalities:

- Barbra Streisand
- Bono (Bono derived his name from a hearing aid store in his hometown of Dublin, Ireland, which had a sign that read "Bonavox Hearing Aids.")
- Cher
- Eric Clapton
- Leonard Nimoy
- Burt Reynolds
- David Suchet
- Pete Townshend
- Myles Kennedy
- Neil Young
- Sylvester Stallone
- Tony Randall
- Sting
- William Shatner (Shatner acquired tinnitus from a loud stage-prop explosion on the set of an episode of *StarTrek*. He says it contributed to the breakup of his second marriage and even made him consider suicide.)
- David Letterman
- Don Imus
- Garrison Keillor
- Larry King
- Peter Jennings
- Phil Collins
- Steve Martin (He acquired tinnitus while filming a pistol-shooting scene in *Three Amigos!* in 1986.)
- Howard Hughes

## Artists, Composers, Writers:

- Vincent van Gogh
- Bedrich Smetana—it was a high E that caused his trouble

- César Franck
- Ludwig van Beethoven (He was driven mad by "rushing and roaring sounds" in his head. "My ears whistle and buzz constantly day and night. I can say I am living a wretched life.")
- Oscar Wilde
- Francisco de Goya
- Robert Schumann

## Historical Figures:
- Charles Darwin
- Dwight D. Eisenhower
- Jean-Jacques Rousseau
- Joan of Arc
- Martin Luther
- Thomas Edison
- Ronald Reagan

## Other Celebrities:
- Alan Shepard
- Cheryl Tiegs
- Jack Straw
- Ted Nugent

Tinnitus is not a disease; it is a symptom resulting from a range of underlying causes:
- Age-associated hearing loss
- Anxiety
- Cerumen (earwax) impaction
- Depression
- Ear infection
- Exposure to excessive or loud noises
- Head injury
- Hearing loss

- High cholesterol
- Jaw misalignment
- Lead poisoning
- Mercury poisoning
- Middle ear infection
- Multiple sclerosis
- Psychedelic drugs
- Sinus infection
- Thyroid disorder
- Vitamin B$_{12}$ deficiency

Tinnitus may have a tonal quality but it is always a simple sound—basically a monotone. In contrast, people with auditory hallucinations hear more complex things that sound like voices singing or music.

Folklore remedies for tinnitus:
- First written account of medical treatment of tinnitus is all the way back to the Egyptians. For the bewitched ear and humming in the ears they would infuse oil, frankincense, tree sap, herbs, and soil; they would administer it via a reed stalk that they put in the external ear.
- The Mesopotamians documented on clay tilework their rituals, and they chanted to get rid of the whispering or singing in the ears.
- Early Greco-Roman medicine defined the treatment of tinnitus based on the cause of the disease so they were the first to really try to relate the two. If the ringing stemmed from a cold, then the ear should be cleaned and the breath held until some humor (body fluid) froths out from it. If the tinnitus stems from the head, then exercise, rubbing, and gargling should be carried out as well as dieting, and placing radish, cucumber juice, honey, and vinegar in the ear.
- Hippocrates and Aristotle were the first to introduce the idea of masking. They were fond of saying "Why

is it that buzzing in the ear ceases if one makes a sound? Is it because a greater sound drives out the less?"

- In the Middle Ages this pouring of things into the ear continued. A Welsh treatment recommended taking a loaf of hot bread, dividing it in two, and putting it in each ear as hot as you could take it and thus perspire, and by the help of God you would be cured.
- In the Renaissance, surgery was used in the treatment of tinnitus. They thought it was wind that was entrapped in the ear and so they put a hole in the mastoid bone to allow the wind to escape.

## Other Information:

Today tinnitus affects many people. It affects 30 percent of the adult population; however, only 6 percent of this 30 percent report incapacitating symptoms. Most of the people who do seek medical care, however, feel that they have been told that there is nothing that can be done about it and that they have to learn to live with it. The prevalence of tinnitus increases with age and has been shown to be independent of noise exposure. It seems to be more common in men, Caucasians, and lower-income families. It has also been seen in children. Thirteen percent of school-age children experience tinnitus.

- Ancient Oriental mysticism regarded tinnitus as sensitivity to the divine.
- Roman medicine associated it with depressive and seizure disorders.
- In the Babylonian Talmud, tinnitus appears as Titus's curse: a gnat buzzing in the brain.
- Pliny the Elder coined the term tinnitus thousands of years ago and the Phoenicians wrote about it.
- Egyptian hieroglyphics depict tinnitus.
- Aristotle noted it in 350 BCE

Tinnitus has also been reported to be a side effect of many prescribed and over-the-counter medications: A list of these include the following:

## Trade/Brand-names

| | | |
|---|---|---|
| Advil | Elavil | Prozac |
| Aleve | Erythromycin | Q-Vel |
| Amikin | Feldene | Rheumatrex |
| Anafranil | Flagyl | Sandimmune |
| Aralen | Gentamicin | Sarafem |
| Aredia | Indocin | Sinequan |
| Aspirin | Intron | Sumycin |
| Biaxin | Lasix | Tobradex |
| Blenoxane | Motrin | Tofranil |
| Bumex | Mustargen | Vancocin |
| Chloromycetin | Naprosyn | Velban |
| Cleocin | Nardil | Viagra |
| Comvax | Neoral | Vincasar |
| Depakene | NSAIDs | Vivactil |
| Depakote | Paraplatin | Wellbutrin |
| Desferal | PEG-Intron | Xylocaine |
| Desyrel | Platinol | Zyban |
| Edecrin | Prograf | |
| Effexor | Propacil | |

# PART E
# NOSE AND SMELL
# DISORDERS

## Introduction (Olfaction)

Smell is the sense of memory and desire.
—Jean-Jacques Rousseau

Smell is often our first response to stimuli. It alerts us to fire before we see flames. It helps us keep safe by helping us choose good foods and avoid those that have gone bad. It makes us recoil before we taste rotten food. Smell, like taste, is a chemical sense detected by sensory cells called *chemoreceptors*. Microscopic molecules released by the substances around us (foods, flowers, smoke, noxious fumes, etc.) stimulate these sensory cells, which pass on electrical impulses to the brain. The brain then interprets patterns in electrical activity as specific odors and olfactory sensation becomes perception—something we can recognize as smell.

"The sense of smell is a primal sense for humans as well as for animals. From an evolutionary standpoint smell is one of

the most ancient of senses. Smell (or olfaction) allows verte-
brates and other organisms with olfactory receptors to identify
food, mates, predators, and provides both sensual pleasure
(the odor of flowers and perfume) as well as warnings of danger." The sense of smell also determines the flavor of the
foods we eat and the beverages we drink. Smells influence our
moods and motivation and hence also our behavior. According
to Greek tradition, the oracle at Delphi put herself in the mood
by inhaling the smell of burning laurel.

Although smell is the most direct and basic of our senses,
it seems to be the sense we take most for granted. But smell,
more so than any other sense, is also intimately linked to the
parts of the brain that process emotion and associative learn-
ing. Smell and taste loss can lead to depression.

The nose is a very complex organ. The human nose has
over ten million receptors of twenty basic types. If your nose
is in maximum working order your brain can interpret the combination of these receptors to recognize any one of between
4,000 and 10,000 different smells.

Even though humans can recognize about 10,000 different
scents, of all the senses, the olfactory sensory faculty is the
least appreciated sense of the human body. To humans, the
sense of smell is not as crucial for survival as it is in animals.
The stronger olfactory senses in other creatures makes it possible for them to find food, water, and shelter through the act
of sniffing. We rely on sight, sound, and dexterity for fundamental survival skills. Bloodhounds can smell an odor that is
a thousand times weaker than one perceptible by humans. At
the most basic level, a smell can be used by a baby to identify
its mother. Although the sense of smell declines as we grow
older, odor memory endures when other remembrances have
grown dim.

Most of us take our sense of smell for granted. Picture a
world without the scent of flowers, the ocean, the smell of
freshly baked bread, newly picked basil, or the aroma of just-
brewed coffee. The senses are important for our total life expe-

rience of emotions and recollections. Smell, in particular, can stir up deep-seated feelings and conjure up powerful memories. There are smells we hate, smells we love, and smells that remind us of certain situations or places. How senseless would it be if you could no longer smell something—like Marcel Proust's famous and redolent *madeleines*—that brought back a favorite memory? Proust glorified the *madeleine* when he wrote, "I raised to my lips a spoonful of the cake . . . a shudder ran through my whole body and I stopped, intent upon the extraordinary changes that were taking place."

It's surprising to learn that flavors are recognized principally through the sense of smell. Along with texture, temperature, and the sensations from the common chemical sense, the perception of flavor comes from a combination of odors and taste. Without the olfactory cells, familiar flavors like coffee or oranges would be harder to distinguish. You couldn't taste anything without some help of the nose. Most of your sense of taste is really about your sense of smell. The ability to smell and taste go hand in hand because odors from food allow us to taste more fully. Taste is 75 percent smell.

Every year, thousands of people develop problems with their sense of smell. More than 200,000 people visit a physician each year for help with smell disorders or related problems. Many people who have smell disorders also notice problems with their sense of taste.

## Types of smell disorders:
- Anosmia—loss of the sense of smell (q.v.)
- Dysosmia—an impairment of the sense of smell
- Euosmia—a pleasant odor
- Hyposmia—reduced ability to detect odors
- Parosmia—distorted sense of smell (q.v.)
- Phantosmia—smelling odors that aren't present
- Troposmia—distorted sense of smell (synonym for parosmia)

Some causes and associations of smell disorders:
- Dental problems
- Diabetes
- Exposure to solvents and insecticides
- Head injuries
- Hormonal disturbances
- Medications (see list on page 206)
- Nasal polyps
- Obesity
- Parkinsonism
- Radiation treatment for head and neck cancers
- Recent illness or injury
- Sinus infections
- Upper respiratory infections (colds, flu)

## Nose Trivia:

One smells more when lying on the ground than when standing because many odors are heavier than air.

Women have a keener sense of smell than men.

"The first sensory perception in our existence, even before our birth, is of a smell contained in the amniotic fluid."

The sixteenth-century philosopher Michel de Montaigne wrote an essay on smells. He considered himself a great smeller—supposedly because of his mustache, which retained smells from the air.

Cyrano de Bergerac, the title character in the popular play by Edmond Rostand, is a brilliant, strong-willed man of many talents, a charismatic swordsman and a remarkable poet. He, however, has an extremely oversized nose, which is a target for his own self-doubt.

Nikolai Gogol: published his short story, "*The Nose*," a grotesque tale about a nose that detaches itself from a major's face and to the major's dismay, insists on leading an independent existence. Dmitri Shostakovich wrote an opera, based on Gogol's story.

# Smell Disturbances

## Loss of Smell

(Anosmia, Odor Blindness, Anosphrasia)

> They haven't got no noses
> The fallen sons of Eve
> Even the smell of roses
> Is not what they supposes
> But more than mind discloses
> And more than men believe.
> —G.K. Chesterton, "The Song of Quoodle"

The term *anosmia* means the total absence of the sense of smell. Anosmics, people suffering from anosmia, are unable to identify scents of any kind. It has been estimated that more than two million people in the United States have a severely damaged smell function to the point that they can smell nothing.

The loss of smell can affect people socially, psychologically, and physiologically. It can lead to loss of self-worth and libido—a good deal of human interaction depends on smell—as well as weight loss or gain, because people with no sense of taste either forget to eat or overcompensate by eating excessively. Anosmia is to smell as blindness is to sight, or as deafness is to hearing.

Among the more than 200 medical conditions that have been reported to cause loss of smell include the following:

- Allergies
- Alzheimer's disease
- Anemia
- Brain tumors
- Diabetes
- Gingivitis

- Glossitis
- Head trauma
- Hypertension
- Influenza
- Malnutrition
- Nasal polyps
- Obesity
- Parkinsonism
- Poor oral hygiene
- Smoking
- Tooth infection
- Upper respiratory infection
- Vitamin $B_{12}$ deficiency
- Yeast infection of the tongue

In addition, the normal aging process can be responsible for loss of smell. By age sixty-five, about 25 percent of people have serious olfactory impairment, and by age eighty the number is 75 percent.

The sense of smell is vital for many reasons:
- A person with no sense of smell is deprived of an important early warning system for the detection of fires, hazardous fumes, leaking gas, and rotten food.
- Anosmics (people suffering from anosmia) are known to skip meals because the appeal for food has been lost, and not eating causes malnutrition and involuntary weight loss.
- Anosmia can also have the opposite effect causing people to overeat to make up for the loss of taste.
- Smell and taste loss can result in depression.
- Smell determines the flavor of foods and the beverages we consume.
- Smell alerts us to offensive body odors.
- Taste and smell are very strongly linked. You can smell without tasting, but your taste is greatly affected if you cannot smell.

- We can smell smoke at concentrations below that needed to activate most sensitive household smoke detectors.

Celebrities who are or were anosmic include the following:
- Ben Cohen (of Ben & Jerry's ice-cream store fame)
- Bill Pullman
- Brian Mulroney
- Justin Hayward
- Karen Duffy
- Michael Hutchence
- Stevie Wonder
- William Wordsworth

Blind people regularly identify other individuals by each person's unique odor. Helen Keller, who grew up blind and deaf, had to depend on her sense of smell for essential information about her surroundings, and found that it became a source of extreme pleasure. She lamented the fact that smell "does not hold the high position it deserves among its sisters," adding, "I doubt if there is any sensation arising from sight more delightful than the odors which filter through sun-warmed, wind-tossed branches, or the tide of scents which swells, subsides, rises again wave on wave, filling the wide world with invisible sweetness." Calling smell the "fallen angel," she claimed that she could judge character by sniffing; a theory has been substantiated by modern scientific studies.

The seventeenth-century poet Robert Herrick wrote a poem called "*Julia's Sweat." Napoleon famously sent Josephine the following erotic line from the thick of battle, *"Je reviens en trois jours; ne te laves pas!"* "I will return in three days. Don't wash!"

London (Reuters)—In March 2008, the Lloyd's of London insurance market has insured the nose of a leading wine maker and taster, Ilja Gort, the Dutch owner of Chateau de la Garde in Bordeaux and producer of Tulipe Wines, for 8 million dollars, covering the Bordeaux producer against the loss of his nose and sense of smell. It is said that his nose could distinguish millions of different scents and was essential to guarantee the quality of his wines.

Certain medications, prescribed and over the counter, can weaken or curtail the sense of smell:

## Trade/Brand-names

| | | |
|---|---|---|
| Adalat | Cipro | Oxsoralen |
| Adoxa | Cold-Eze | Procardia |
| Amoxil | Cordarone | Ruxid |
| Augmentin | Cosopt | Streptomycin |
| Biaxin | Kantrex | Trusopt |
| Celexa | Monodox | Zicam |

*Julia's Sweat*
by Robert Herrick
Would ye oil of blossoms get?
Take it from my Julia's sweat:
Oil of lilies and of spike?
From her moisture take the like,
Let her breathe, or let her blow,
All rich spices thence will flow.

## Sneezing

(Sternutation)

If you sneeze on Monday you sneeze for
   danger,
Sneeze on Tuesday, kiss a stranger,
Sneeze on Wednesday, sneeze for a
   letter,
Sneeze on Thursday, something better,

Sneeze on Friday, sneeze for sorrow,
Sneeze on Saturday, see your sweet-
heart tomorrow.

Sneezing, like coughing, is a natural defense mechanism of the body for clearing irritants, toxins, or foreign substances from the nose. It is an involuntary, audible expulsion of air through the nose and mouth. Sneezing, also known as *sternutation*, was once considered to be the body driving out evil spirits. Today we know that the sudden forceful ejection of air through the nose and mouth is caused by irritation of the mucous membrane. Normally, people sneeze once or twice during early morning or during the day to clear the nose.

Sneezing involves contraction of the muscles of the face, neck, and eyes. When we sneeze, the protective reflex of the eyes causes our eyes to squeeze shut. An urban legend states that you cannot open your eyes while you sneeze, or if you manage to your eyes will pop out. During a sneeze the impulses travel through your face causing your eyelids to blink; this response is entirely automatic.

The reason behind the powerful nature of a sneeze is its involvement of not simply the nose and mouth, but numerous organs of the upper body—it is a response that involves the muscles of the face, throat, and chest. In recent years, studies have shown that stifling or holding back sneezes can cause damage to the sinuses as well as to the inner ear and brain cells resulting in tinnitus (ringing in the ears), reduced high-frequency hearing, and rupturing the ear drum.

Sneezing is the body's way of removing irritants. Almost anything that irritates the nose can provoke a sneezing fit. Allergic people also sneeze because they release irritant chemicals into the nose when they come into contact with allergens like pollens, dust mites, or animals. It begins with irritation of the lining of the nose, and ends in an explosion of air from the nose and mouth.

During sneezing, secretions of the nose are being expelled as droplets (about 40,000) up to ten feet away. When these droplets contain contagious bacteria and viruses, they spread infection throughout the area of droplets sprayed. The material spread by sneezing can travel at a speed of around 100 miles per hour—a great way to spread germs.

Symptoms associated with sneezing include the following:
- Breathlessness
- Bursting type of headache
- Disturbed sleep
- Dizziness
- General body aches
- Hoarseness
- Lack of concentration
- Loss of smell
- Nasal speech
- Nausea
- Poor appetite
- Restlessness
- Ringing in ears (q.v.)
- Sore throat
- Vomiting
- Watery and itching nose

Causes of sneezing include any or all of the following:
- Allergic reactions to a variety of substances
- Bacterial and viral infections (the common cold or flu)
- Carpets, pillows, mattresses, rugs, furry and stuffed toys
- Certain types of fungal infection
- Chilies, cucumber, watermelon as well as fish, meat, and egg
- Cold weather, rain water, dampness, and temperature variations

- Contact with animals—dander and mites of cats, dogs, and birds
- Foods, preservatives, and food coloring
- Herbs—plants, grass, trees, and pollens
- Irritants—smoke, pollution, pollens, pepper, powders, pesticides, insecticides, and dusts
- Mechanically plucking hair in the nose
- Combing hair, tweezing eyebrows, rubbing the inner corner of the eye, and even by eating too much.

Have you ever emerged from a matinee movie, squinted into the sudden burst of sunlight and sneezed uncontrollably? One in every three people will answer this question with an emphatic "Yes." In certain individuals, sneezing can be triggered by sudden exposure to bright light, particularly that of the sun. This response is known as the "photic" sneeze reflex.

**Trivia:**
- A twelve-year-old girl named Donna Griffiths, from England, holds the longest attack of sneezing on record. Donna was reported to have sneezed for over 977 days between January 1981 and September 1983. Their frequency was, at first, every minute. As the days moved into weeks and years her sneezes became less frequent and occurred about every five minutes.
- Some cultures have considered sneezing a sign of good fortune, whereas others have seen it as an omen of death. The saying "God bless you" is thought to have emerged during the Bubonic Plague of the sixth century, where sneezing was one of its early symptoms.
- In the Hellenistic cultures of Classical Antiquity, sneezes were believed to be prophetic signs from the gods. In 410 BCE, the Athenian general

Xenophon strongly urged his fellow soldiers to follow him to liberty or to death against the Persians. He spoke for an hour inspiring his army and guaranteeing them a safe return to Athens at which time a soldier emphasized his conclusion with a sneeze. Thinking that this sneeze was a favorable sign from the gods, the soldiers bowed before Xenophon and followed his command.

- In the early Middle Ages, it was believed that one's life was in fact tied to one's breath—a belief reflected in the word "expire" (originally meaning "to exhale"), gaining the additional meaning of "to come to an end" or "to die." The significant amount of breath expelled from the body during a sneeze, had likely led people to believe that sneezing could easily be fatal.

- The Japanese attach significance to the number of times a man sneezes. Thus, one sneeze indicates that someone is praising him, while two can be a sign of censure or disparagement; a triple sneeze is commonplace and means simply that a person has caught a cold.

- In Scotland even educated people have been known to maintain that idiots are incapable of sneezing. If this is true, the inference is clear that the act of sternutation is indisputable evidence of the possession of a certain degree of intelligence.

- British nurses used to think that infants were under a fairy spell until they sneezed.

- Among some peoples, the sneeze of a young child has a certain mystic significance, and is intimately associated with its prospective welfare or bad luck. When, therefore, a Maori infant sneezes, its mother immediately recites a long charm of words. If the sneeze occurs during a meal, it is thought to be prognostic of a visit or of some interesting piece of news; whereas in Tonga it is deemed an evil token.

- So, too, among the New Zealanders, if a child sneezes on the occasion of receiving its name, the officiating priest at once holds to its ear the wooden image of an idol and sings some mystic words.
- In Turkistan, when a person to whom a remark is addressed sneezes, it is a declaration that the opinion or statement is correct, just as if the person accosted were to exclaim, "That is true!" In the same country three sneezes are unlucky. When, also, any one hiccoughs, it is etiquette to say, "You stole something from me," and this phrase at such times is supposed to produce good luck.
- It was a Flemish belief that a sneeze during a conversation proved that what one said was the truth, a doctrine which must have commended itself to snuff-takers.
- According to a Chinese superstition, a sneeze on New Year's Eve is ominous for the coming year; to offset this, the sneezer must visit three families of different surnames and beg from each a small tortoise-shaped cake, which must be eaten before midnight.
- People from Sussex are prejudiced against cats, which develop sneezing proclivities, for they believe that, when a pet feline sneezes thrice, it augurs ill for the health of the household, and is premonitory of influenza and bronchial affections.
- In Shetlandic and Welsh folklore the sneeze of a cat indicates cold north winds in summer and snow in winter.
- Cat folklore in Italy says that a cat sneezing is supposed to be a good omen for everyone who hears it. Other superstitions say that a cat sneezing once means there will be rain; that if a cat sneezes three times, the family will catch a cold; and that a sneezing cat is a sign of future wealth.

- Pope Gregory the Great, in response to the sixth-century plague in Italy, regarded the sneeze as a sure sign of approaching sickness. He is responsible for insisting that prayers, such as "God bless you!" be said in response to the deadly sneeze.
- It is written in the Talmud that the patriarch Jacob was the first person to actually become ill before passing on. Before that, people would sneeze and die. When God infused the soul into Man, He "blew it" into Adam's nostrils. Thus, when it came time for the soul to be returned to its Maker, it would leave through the same portal it arrived.
- Primitive people held the belief that a sneeze signified approaching death, and immediately assisted the distressed person by crying out "God help you!" Egyptians, Romans, and Greeks saw the sneeze as an omen of approaching danger, or, on a more positive note, as a way of foretelling the future.
- *Snatiation* is a medical disorder characterized by uncontrollable bursts of sneezing brought on by fullness of the stomach, and typically observed in sufferers immediately after a large meal.
- It is not possible to urinate during a sneezing spasm.

Medications that have been reported to cause an attack of sneezing include the following:

## Trade/Brand-names

| | | |
|---|---|---|
| Aceon | Bentyl | Pancrease |
| Actifed | Chlor-Trimeton | Rhinocort |
| Aeroid | Claritin | Robitussin |
| Alamast | Cytoxan | Simulect |
| Alomide | Ethyol | Sudafed |
| Astelin | Flomax | Synarel |
| Axert | Gastrocrom | Thiopental |
| Azactam | Gastrografin | Ultravist |
| Beconase | Kinevac | Vicodin |

# PART F
# TASTE AND TASTE
# DISORDERS

Taste *(gustation)* is the weakest of the traditional five senses. It refers to the ability to detect the flavor of substances such as food and poisons. In humans the sense of taste combines with the sense of smell in the perception of flavor. In Western culture, we describe five basic tastes: bitter, salty, sour, sweet, and *umami.* Our taste cells can identify five main qualities: bitter, salty, sour, sweet, and umami. Umami, a fundamental taste in Chinese and Japanese cooking, is the name for the taste sensation produced by compounds such as *glutamate*— (actually glutamic acid or MSG)—and are commonly found in fermented and aged foods. Sometimes described as "meaty" or "savory," or "brothy," the word comes from the Japanese word that means "delicious flavor." Examples of food with the umami taste are parmesan and Roquefort cheese, soy sauce, and fish sauce. It is also found in significant amounts in various foods such as walnuts, grapes, broccoli, tomatoes, and mushrooms. The glutamate taste sensation is most intense in combination with table salt. This is one reason why tomatoes exhibit a stronger taste after adding salt. Sauces with umami and salty tastes are very popular for cooking, such as tomato sauces and ketchup for Western cuisines and soy sauce and fish sauce for East Asian and Southeast Asian cuisines.

Taste is a sensory function of the central nervous system. The receptor cells for taste—taste buds—are found primarily on the surface of the tongue and along the soft palate. The average adult has approximately 10,000 taste buds; children have more. This is one of the reasons that infants and children are very sensitive to different foods. In general, girls have more taste buds than boys do.

Our brain then tells us what flavors we actually taste. Smell also increases our enjoyment of practically everything we eat. Much of what we commonly refer to as "flavor" is actually a combination of smell and taste, with taste most often assuming the secondary position.

The various tastes are:
- Bitterness. Bitter taste is perceived by many to be unpleasant, sharp, or disagreeable. Common bitter foods and beverages include coffee, unsweetened chocolate, beer, some olives, citrus peel, dandelion greens, and escarole. Quinine, found in tonic water, is also known for its bitter taste.
- Saltiness. Saltiness is a taste produced primarily by the presence of sodium ions.
- Sourness. Sourness is the taste that detects acidity.
- Sweetness. Sweetness is produced by the presence of sugars, some proteins, and a few other substances.
- Umami (see above)

Many factors affect taste perception, including some medical conditions such as:
- Aging
- Color/vision impairments
- Hormonal influences
- Genetic variations
- Oral temperature
- Drugs and chemicals
- Brain tumors
- Stuffed noses
- Zinc deficiency
- Viral infections

## Taste Bud Trivia:
- The tongue has about 10,000 taste buds, each having ten to fifteen receptacles that send messages to the brain.
- Over a two-week period, the body generates an entire new set of taste buds, which continues until we reach our seventies and eighties. Onions and garlic, alcohol, caffeine, hot and spicy foods, and smoking dull the taste buds. It takes about a day for taste buds to cleanse themselves after being exposed to these substances.
- Taste buds are most sensitive right after a night's sleep.
- Insects have taste organs on their feet, antennae, and mouth parts. Fish can taste with their fins and tail as well as their mouth

## Loss of Taste

### (Ageusia)

*Ageusia*, also called *taste blindness* or gustatory anesthesia, is the complete loss of taste functions of the tongue. It is the inability to distinguish sweet, sour, bitter, or salty substances. Most of what is perceived as the sense of taste is in fact acquired from smell. Approximately 25 percent of Americans are nontasters.

Some people can taste but their ability to do so is diminished. This reduced sensitivity to detect any variations in gustatory sensation is known as *hypogeusia*. *Dysgeusia* denotes a perversion or alteration of taste. (q.v.)

Taste loss can arise as a result of the following conditions:
- Aging
- Brain tumor
- Cancer
- Facial fractures
- Head and brain injury

- Heavy smoking
- High-altitude headache
- Kidney failure
- Leprosy
- Liver failure
- Multiple sclerosis
- Myasthenia gravis
- Vitamin B$_3$ deficiency
- Zinc deficiency

Taste loss is often a complication of *Bell's palsy*, a paralysis of the facial nerve resulting in the inability to control facial muscles on the affected side.

Celebrities who have been affected by Bell's palsy:

- Curtis LeMay
- George Clooney
- Jamey Sheridan
- Jane Greer
- Pierce Brosnan
- Ralph Kiner
- Ralph Nader
- Roseanne Barr

Various medications that have been known to cause taste loss include the following:

### Trade/Brand-names

| | | |
|---|---|---|
| Accutane | Clinoril | Fungizone |
| Adriamycin | Cozaar | Gris-Peg |
| Aralen | Depen | Ismotic |
| Arava | Dilantin | Lamisil |
| Atacand | Effexor | Lincocin |
| Baclofen | Flagyl | Mycobutin |
| Capoten | Flexeril | Nitrodur |

Trade/Brand-names

| | | |
|---|---|---|
| Plavix | Tapazole | Vasotec |
| Precose | Tegretol | Zestril |
| Prinivil | Trancopal | |

## Distorted Taste

(Dysgeusia)

> Smell and taste are in fact but a single
> composite sense, whose laboratory is
> the mouth and its chimney the nose . . .
> —Anthelme Brillat-Savarin

*Dysgeusia* is a persistent distorted or perverted sense of taste. It is often used to describe any change—bad, metallic, salty, rancid, or merely foul—that affects the ability to taste. The sense of taste is frequently dulled or impaired due to a dysfunction of the sense of smell. Our taste buds are filled with specialized cells that collect taste information, which is sent to the brain. Approximately 75 percent of flavor and taste sensations come from nerve cells involved with smell. In some people with dysgeusia, the sense of smell can also be distorted. Both taste and smell cells work together to generate the sense of taste.

Severe long standing dysgeusia can be clinically significant as it may lead to individuals losing interest in food. This altered dietary intake creates nutritional deficiencies that may exacerbate pre-existing disease or trigger new ones.

Dysgeusia is relatively common and can have numerous causes, many of which are temporary. For example, the common cold, flu, a nasal or sinus infection, strep throat, and other short-term conditions can cause mild dysgeusia. A list of possible causes of distorted taste include the following:

- Aging
- Bell's palsy
- Brain tumor or trauma to the head
- Burning mouth syndrome
- Cancer
- Copper deficiency
- Cushing's Syndrome
- Damage to the taste nerves
- Depression
- Diabetes
- Dry mouth (xerostomia) (q.v.)
- Gingivitis
- Glossitis
- Head and neck radiation
- Hypothyroidism
- Inflammation of the tongue (glossitis)
- Influenza
- Liver or kidney failure
- Mercury poisoning
- Migraine headache
- Multiple sclerosis
- Nasal polyps
- Radiation therapy
- Respiratory infections such as colds, sinus infections, and throat infections
- Smoking
- Strep throat
- Stroke
- Surgery of the larynx (voice box)
- Thyroid disease
- Vitamin or mineral deficiency

A metallic taste also may be caused by a substance present in the mouth. Medications that are chewed, rather than swallowed, may cause a temporary metallic taste at the back of the tongue.

Medications associated with distorted taste include the following:

## Trade/Brand-names

| | | |
|---|---|---|
| Adalat | Hibiclens | Plavix |
| Adderall | Hyzaar | Precose |
| Adriamycin | Ketek | Prilosec |
| Asacol | Lamictal | Procardia |
| Aspirin | Lamisil | Protonix |
| Atacand | Lasix | Rheumatrex |
| Biaxin | Levsinex | Rhinocort |
| Brethine | Lincocin | Ridaura |
| Capoten | Lioresal | Robitussin |
| Cardizem | Maxalt | Rocephin |
| Cozaar | Monopril | Sinemet |
| Cytoxan | Myambutol | SPRYCEL |
| Depen | Neoral | Tegretol |
| Desoxyn | Neosar | Tetracyclines |
| Diamox | Nexium | Tiazac |
| Didronel | Nitrodur | Topamax |
| Diflucan | Noroxin | Trancopal |
| Edecrin | Oral contraceptives | Vincasar |
| Emend | Paraplatin | Vitamin K |
| Ergocalciferol | Pepcid | Zithromax |
| Flagyl | Persantine | Zyloprim |
| Fungizone | Plaquenil | |

# PART G
# MISCELLANEOUS
# REACTION
# PATTERNS

## Color Blindness

(Dyschromatopsia; Impaired Color Vision)

*Dyschromatopsia* is a visual defect resulting in the inability to distinguish colors. People afflicted more often than not have excellent vision, but they tend to see colors in a limited range of hues. Many of those who suffer this disorder cannot tell the difference between shades of red and green. Achromatopsia, which is exceedingly rare, refers to the total inability to see any colors. People affected by this observe the world in shades of gray and are extremely sensitive to light.

Most of the time, color blindness, occurring in about 8 percent of men and less than 1 percent of women, is caused by an inherited trait; less commonly, it occurs as part of the aging process or is brought about by disease—disorders of the retina or the optic nerve or from certain degenerative disorders of the eyes as well as various chronic illnesses. These include the following:

- Accidents or strokes that damage the retina or affect particular areas of the brain
- Alzheimer's disease

- Chronic alcoholism
- Diabetes
- Glaucoma
- Leukemia
- Liver disease
- Macular degeneration
- Multiple sclerosis
- Parkinsonism
- Retinitis pigmentosa
- Sickle cell anemia

Occupational exposure to certain chemicals can lead to color blindness. This is usually classified as a disability. Industrial or environmental chemicals such as carbon monoxide, carbon disulfide, fertilizers, styrene, and some containing lead can cause loss of color vision.

Various medications have been implicated in the development of color blindness. Some art historians have suggested that the prevalent use of yellow in the work of the famous artist Vincent van Gogh (1853–1890) may have been a result of digitalis, which van Gogh may have ingested as a treatment for epilepsy.

Drugs reported to cause eye color changes include the following:

## Trade/Brand-names

| | | |
|---|---|---|
| Aralen | Dilantin | Plaquenil |
| Cialis | Heroin | Rifamate |
| Cordarone | Lamisil | Sabril |
| Depakene | Lanoxin | Tegretol |
| Depakote | Levitra | Viagra |
| Desferal | Myambutol | |

# Flatulence

## (Farting)

*Flatulence* is the state of having excessive stomach or intestinal gas. It is the presence of a mixture of gases in the digestive tract—the esophagus, stomach, small intestine, and large intestine—of mammals. Such a mixture of gases is known as flatus; this is expelled from the rectum in a process colloquially known as "farting," among other terms. The unpleasant odor often associated with flatus is generally attributed to sulfur-containing compounds, produced only by particular bacteria not found in everyone. Flatulence itself, although not life threatening, can definitely cause social embarrassment.

Everyone passes gas normally each day. A certain amount of gas is present in your gastrointestinal tract at any one time, mainly in your stomach and colon. Most people produce about one to three pints a day and pass gas about fourteen times a day; up to twenty to twenty-five times is considered normal. More than that may be excessive. Gas in the digestive tract comes from swallowed air and the normal breakdown of certain undigested foods by harmless bacteria naturally present in the large intestine.

The noises commonly associated with flatulence are caused by the vibration of the anal sphincter, and occasionally by the closed buttocks. The sound varies depending on the tightness of the sphincter muscle and velocity of the gas being propelled, as well as other factors such as water and body fat. Among humans, flatulence sometimes happens accidentally, as does coughing or sneezing; but flatulence can be voluntarily elicited by tensing the rectum or "bearing down" and subsequently releasing the anal sphincter, resulting in the expulsion of a flatus. Humans are also known to flatulate during sleep, largely due to the relaxed state of body muscles, which results in the average person flatulating about ten to twenty times through any given night.

Foods that produce gas in one person may not cause gas in another. Some common bacteria in the large intestine can destroy the hydrogen that other bacteria produce. The balance of the two types of bacteria may explain why some people have more gas than others. Most foods that consist of carbohydrates can cause gas. By contrast, fats and proteins cause little gas.

Flatulence-producing foods include beans, lentils, dairy products, onions, garlic, scallions, leeks, radishes, sweet potatoes, cashews, Jerusalem artichokes, oats, wheat, yeast in breads, starches, red wine, dark beer, foods containing soluble and insoluble fiber and others. Cauliflower, broccoli, cabbage, and other cruciferous vegetables are commonly reputed to not only increase flatulence, but to increase the pungency of the flatus.

In addition to causing embarrassment and unease, flatulence is linked to a variety of symptoms, some of which may be distressing and may herald the onset of significant gastrointestinal diseases or may represent functional bowel disorders.

In many cultures, human flatulence in public is regarded as embarrassing and repulsive, even to the point of being a taboo subject. People will often strain to hold in the passing of gas when in polite company, or position themselves to conceal the noise and smell. In other cultures it may be no more embarrassing than coughing.

Flatulence is a potential source of humor, either due to the foul smell or the sounds produced. Some find humor in flatulent ignition (also called "pyroflatulence"), which is possible due to the presence of flammable gases such as hydrogen and methane, though the process can result in burn injuries to the rectum, anus, and surrounding buttocks.

While the act of bypassing flatus is generally considered to be a disgraceful occurrence in public settings, flatulence may, in casual circumstances, be used as either a humorous addition to a joke, or as a comic occurrence in and of itself.

In *The City of God,* St. Augustine, not otherwise noted for his levity, makes mention of men who "have such command of their bowels, that they can break wind continuously at will, so as to produce the effect of singing."

In the mid-1800s, flatulence took center stage with the French entertainer Joseph Pugol ("Le Pétomane"). Pugol, "the Fartiste," was able to pass gas at will and at varying pitch. He did flatulence impressions and played tunes for sold-out shows at the Moulin Rouge. The performer Mr. Methane carries on Le Pétomane's tradition even today.

Bulgaria regularly holds annual Flatulence competitions, based on Internet votes. The winner in 2006 and 2007 was a famous Mafia-linked personality called Maria Doychinova. Local media suggested, rather unkindly, that her bad breath was actually worse than her flatulence.

Although it is likely that flatulence humor has long been considered amusing in cultures that consider the public passing of gas impolite, such jokes are rarely recorded. An important early text is the fifth century BCE play, *The Knights,* by Aristophanes which has numerous fart jokes.

In the translated version of Penguin's *1001 Arabian Nights Tales*, a story entitled "The Historic Fart" tells of a man that flees his country from the sheer embarrassment of farting at his wedding.

One of the most celebrated incidences of flatulence humor in early English literature is in *The Miller's Tale* by Geoffrey Chaucer, which dates from the fourteenth century. The character Nicholas hangs his buttocks out of a window and farts in the face of his rival Absolom. Absolom then sears Nicholas's backside with a red-hot poker.

François Rabelais' *Gargantua and Pantagruel* is laden with acts of flatulence. In Chapter XXVII of the second book, the giant, Pantagruel, releases a fart that "made the earth shake for twenty-nine miles around, and the foul air he blew out created more than fifty-three thousand tiny men, dwarves, and creatures of weird shapes, and then he emitted a fat wet fart that turned into just as many tiny stooping women."

Benjamin Franklin, in his open letter "To the Royal Academy of Farting," satirically proposes that converting farts into a more agreeable form through science should be a milestone goal of the Royal Academy. "My Prize Question therefore should be, To discover some Drug wholesome & not disagreeable, to be mixed with our common Food, or Sauces, that shall render the natural Discharges of Wind from our Bodies, not only inoffensive, but agreeable as Perfumes."

Mark Twain wrote a one-act play, *1601*, now commonly known as *A Fart in Queen Elizabeth's Court.*

Flatulence humor and the lighting of farts also appear in cinema and television. Farting featured heavily in one scene of *Blazing Saddles*. This caused some controversy in the United States when it was run as a television movie of the week by ABC, the farting sounds were overdubbed with sounds from the surrounding horses, so the scene had cowboys sitting around a campfire standing up and leaning over for no apparent reason. *Star Trek V*, the first and only Star Trek production to contain a fart joke, is known jokingly as Blazing Starships in reference to the bean-eating cowboys in *Blazing Saddles*.

"I fart in your general direction" is a popular phrase from *Monty Python and the Holy Grail.*

In the movie *Dumb and Dumber*, Lloyd Christmas, played by Jim Carrey, lights a fart during a dream sequence.

Whoopee cushion: A whoopee cushion, also known as a poo-poo cushion and Razzberry Cushion, is a practical joke device that produces a noise resembling a raspberry or human flatulence. It is made from two sheets of rubber that are glued together at the edges. There is a small opening with a flap at one end for air to enter and leave the cushion. To use it, one must first inflate it with air and then place it on a chair. An unsuspecting victim sits on the whoopee cushion, forcing the air out of the opening, which causes the flap to vibrate and produce its distinctive sound. The whoopee cushion has been put to use in numerous books and TV shows.

*The Gas We Pass: The Story of Farts* is a children's book written by Shinta Cho. The book tells children about flatulence, and that it is completely natural to do so. *Everyone Poops* is a prequel. The book also tells us about other animals, and their habits of flatulence. The book also relates why farts smell bad, and what animals only seem to fart (skunks and stink bugs).

History has numerous anecdotal accounts of flatulence; Hippocrates himself professed, that passing gas is necessary to well-being.

The Roman Emperor Claudius decreed that "all Roman citizens shall be allowed to pass gas whenever necessary." Unfortunately for flatulent Romans, Emperor Constantine, in a 315 BCE edict, later reversed this decision.

Drugs that have been known to cause flatulence include the following:

## Trade/Brand-names

| | | |
|---|---|---|
| Aceon | Avelox | Cubicin |
| Aciphex | Axid | Cytotec |
| Actonel | Betapace | Daypro |
| Adalat | Campral | Depakene |
| Adriamycin | Camptosar | Depakote |
| Aggrenox | Carafate | Didronel |
| Aleve | Cardura | Diovan |
| Alina | Casodex | Dipentum |
| Aloxi | Celebrex | Ditropan |
| Ambien | CellCept | Dolobid |
| Amitiza | Chantix | Dostinex |
| Amoxapine | Cipro | Duragesic |
| Amoxil | Claritin | Eldepryl |
| Ampicillin | Clinoril | Elmiron |
| Anafranil | Cognex | Emend |
| Ansaid | Colazal | Estrogens |
| Aptivus | Colestid | Evista |
| Arava | Comtan | Exelon |
| Asacol | Coumadin | Exovac |
| Avapro | Cozaar | Factive |

## Trade/Brand-names

| | | |
|---|---|---|
| Famvir | Monopril | Requip |
| Fiorinal | Motrin | Rhinocort |
| Flagyl | Mycobutin | Rifadin |
| Flecainide | Nalfon | Rilutek |
| Flexeril | Neoral | Rythmol |
| Floxin | Neurontin | Salagen |
| Fosamax | Nexium | Sandostatin |
| Foscavir | Nicoderm | Sectral |
| Fungizone | Nicotine | Simulect |
| Gastrocrom | Nipent | Skelid |
| Geocillin | Noctec | Strattera |
| Gleevec | Noroxin | Suboxone |
| Glucophage | Norpace | Sular |
| Glucotrol | Norvasc | Sutent |
| Glyset | Numorphan | Tarceva |
| Gold | Nutropin | Targretin |
| Hepsera | Omnicef | Tasmar |
| Hyzaar | Orudis | Tensilon |
| Imodium | OxyContin | Teveten |
| Indocin | Paxil | Thalidomid |
| Innohep | Pepto-Bismol | Ticlid |
| Intron A | Pitressin | Tolectin |
| Invanz | Plendil | Topamax |
| Invirase | Pletal | Toprol |
| Ketek | Ponstel | Toradol |
| Lamictal | Precose | Tricor |
| Lexapro | Prevacid | Trizivir |
| Lipitor | Prezista | Tylenol |
| Lodine | Prilosec | Tysabri |
| Luvox | Proamatine | Ultracet |
| Lyrica | Prograf | Ultram |
| Macrobid | ProSom | Valstar |
| Meridia | Protonix | Vascase |
| Meronem | Provigil | Vicodin |
| Mevacor | Prozac | Videx |
| Miacalcin | Rapamune | Viracept |
| Micardis | Relafen | Viread |
| Mobic | Reminyl | Vitamin $B_3$ |

## Trade/Brand-names

| | | |
|---|---|---|
| Voltaren | Zestril | Zosyn |
| Welchol | Ziac | Zyban |
| Wellbutrin | Zithromax | Zyflo |
| Xyrem | Zocor | Zyprexa |
| Zavesca | Zoladex | Zyrtec |
| Zenapax | Zoloft | |
| Zelnorm | Zonegran | |

# Goosebumps

(Cutis Anserina)

Goosebumps, temporary rumpling of the skin into tiny bumps, also called "goose pimples," "gooseflesh," "goose skin," "the creeps," "chill bumps," "chicken skin," "the shivers," or technically, *cutis anserina,* are the bumps on a person's skin at the base of body hairs that develop when a person is cold or experiences strong emotions such as fear or awe. The reflex of producing goosebumps is known as *piloerection* or the *pilomotor reflex*. The words used to describe this condition are curious and colorful. A fancier term for this familiar phenomenon is *horripilation*. Horripilation was compounded from the Latin *horrere.* Goosebumps occur not only in humans but also in other mammals; for example, porcupines raise their quills when threatened.

In response to cold or certain emotional states, such as fear or rage, the smooth muscles of the subsurface layer (dermis) of skin tend to contract, causing the skin to pucker and body hair to stand erect. In furred animals this can serve two purposes, first; erection of the fur may make an animal seem larger than it actually is and act to frighten away a potential aggressor, as noted in frightened cats, and second, the erect fur traps a blanket of air close to the skin, thus providing the animal with additional insulation against loss of body heat.

Goosebumps are strongest on the forearms, but also occur on the legs, back, and other areas of the skin that have hair. In some people, they even occur in the face or on the head.

Piloerection is also a rare symptom of some diseases:
- Temporal lobe epilepsy
- Brain tumors
- Hyperreflexia (abnormally increased reflex action)
- Heroin withdrawal
- Described during seizures

Goosebumps can occur only in mammals, since other animals do not have hair. The term "goosebumps" is therefore misleading: the bumps on the skin of a plucked goose technically do not qualify as piloerection even though this is where the term comes from. Birds do however have a similar reflex of raising their feathers in order to keep warm.

In other languages, the "goose" may be replaced by other kinds of poultry. For instance, "hen" is used in French (*la chair de poule*), and "chicken" is used in Dutch (*Kippenvel*), Spanish (*la piel de gallina*), and Afrikaans (*Grillers*).

Drugs that have been reported to cause goosebumps include the following:

### Trade/Brand-names

| | | |
|---|---|---|
| Dolophine | Ismelin | Proamatine |
| Gabitril | Methadone | Talwin |
| Heroin | Nicoderm | Yohimbine |
| Intropin | Nicotine | |

## Gynecomastia

### (Breast Enlargement in Males)

Gynecomastia is the development of abnormally large *mammary glands* in males resulting in breast enlargement, which can sometimes cause secretion of milk. The term comes from the Greek words *gyne* meaning "woman" and *mastos* denoting "breast." In practical terms, this means abnormally large breasts on men. The condition can occur normally in newborns, in adolescents, and in the elderly.

The condition is relatively common in adolescent boys, and 90 percent of the time symptoms disappear in a matter of months, or, as adolescence wanes, a few years later. Persistence is uncommon in men older than seventeen years. But the remaining 10 percent are tormented with a social handicap that gives rise to a deep and complex shame, and puts a young man's relationship with his body at risk. During puberty, gynecomastia can make boys a target for taunting from their peers. It can make activities like swimming or changing for gym class a traumatic experience. For men, enlarged breasts can be stressful and embarrassing. Gynecomastia can be difficult to hide and a challenge to romantic relationships.

The cause of common gynecomastia has generally been attributed to an imbalance of sex hormones estrogen and testosterone: more estrogen, less testosterone. Most people think of estrogen as an exclusively female hormone, but men also produce it—though normally in small quantities. It helps regulate bone density, sperm production and mood. But male estrogen levels that are too high, or are out of balance with testosterone levels, can lead to gynecomastia.

Signs and symptoms of gynecomastia include the following:

- Breast tenderness
- Nipple discharge
- Swollen breast gland tissue
- Swollen nipples (especially in adolescent boys)

While many cases of gynecomastia have no apparent cause, there are several potential causes and associations of this disorder:

- Aging (Hormone changes that occur with normal aging can cause gynecomastia, especially in men who are overweight.)
- Castration
- Chronic liver disease
- Genetic disorders
- HIV (The human immunodeficiency virus that causes AIDS can cause gynecomastia. Some medications used in the treatment of HIV also can cause gynecomastia.)
- Hyperthyroidism (In this condition, the thyroid gland produces too much of the hormone thyroxine. This can lead to alterations in testosterone and estrogen that cause gynecomastia.)
- Kidney failure
- Liver failure and cirrhosis (In male alcoholics, failure of the liver to inactivate circulating estrogen, as in alcoholic cirrhosis, is a common cause of gynecomastia.)
- Marijuana use
- Obesity
- Puberty
- Starvation
- Steroid abuse ("bitch tits")
- Tumors (Some tumors, usually involving the testicles, adrenal glands, pituitary, lung, and liver, can produce hormones that alter the male-female hormone balance.)

Medications cause about 20 percent of cases of gynecomastia in post-adolescent males. The following drugs have been reported to cause gynecomastia:

## Trade/Brand-names

| | | |
|---|---|---|
| Abilify | Lupron | Rexitene |
| Aciphex | Matulane | Rifamate |
| Adalat | Mevacor | Sandostatin |
| Aldactone | Midamor | Serpasil |
| Aldomet | Mifeprex | Serzone |
| Anafranil | Minipress | Sporanox |
| Androgel | Moban | SPRYCEL |
| Android | Monopril | Stelazine |
| Android-F | Morphine | Sular |
| Avodart | MS Contin | Sustiva |
| Axid | Myleran | Tagamet |
| Azilect | Navane | Tenuate |
| Calan | Neoral | Testosterone |
| Capoten | Nexavar | Thalidomide |
| Cardizem | Nexium | Thorazine |
| Casodex | Nilandron | Tofranil |
| Catapres | Nizoral | Trecator-SC |
| Clinoril | Norpace | Trelstar |
| Compazine | Norvasc | Tricor |
| Cordarone | Nutropin | Trilafon |
| Elavil | Orudis | Trizivir |
| Emcyt | Pamelor | Vantas |
| Eulexin | Phenergan | Vasotec |
| Geodon | Plendil | Vitamin B$_3$ |
| Haldol | Pravachol | Vivactil |
| Inapsine | Prevacid | Wellbutrin |
| Indocin | Prezista | Xanax |
| Inspra | Prilosec | Zocor |
| Lanoxin | Prolixin | Zoloft |
| Lescol | Proscar | Zonegran |
| Lipitor | Prozac | Zyban |
| Loxitane | Reglan | Zyloprim |
| Lunesta | Requip | Zyprexa |

## Hiccoughs

(Singultus)

> A one-year-old baby looks and sounds
> cute with the hiccups.
> —*Leondoni's Magical Creations – 14*
> *Happy Ways to Cure Hiccups*

Hiccoughs, a frequent and mildly annoying disorder, is the result of involuntary, unintentional spasmodic contraction of the diaphragm followed by rapid closure of the vocal cords and trachea. The sudden rush of air into the lungs causes the epiglottis to close, producing the characteristic "hic." Hiccups serve no known physiologic function.

In the seventeenth-century, hiccough was known as a "drunken man's cough," and so became "hiccough," with no change in pronunciation. That spelling became so widespread that Samuel Johnson, in his dictionary, incorrectly wrote that "hiccup" was a perverted form of "hiccough." Francis Bacon (1626) provided the first example of "hiccough" in the Oxford English Dictionary, writing that it had been "observed by the Ancients, that Sneezing doth cease the Hiccough."

The technical term for hiccoughs is singultus. Hiccoughs can develop as a result of the following:

- Belching
- Coughing
- Crying out loud (sobbing causes air to enter the stomach)
- Drinking alcoholic beverages to excess
- Drinking carbonated beverages
- Eating too quickly
- Eating very hot or spicy food
- Long and unrestrained laughter
- Smoking
- Taking a cold drink while eating a hot meal

It is reported that 30 percent of chemotherapy patients suffer hiccoughs as a side effect of treatment. Ultrasound scans have also shown that babies in utero experience hiccups.

Various underlying disease processes have been associated with chronic or intractable hiccoughs:

• Central nervous system maladies
• Chemotherapy (Thirty percent of patients
  undergoing chemotherapy suffer hiccups as a side
  effect of treatment.)
• Diabetes
• Eardrum inflammation
• Early Parkinsonism
• Gastrointestinal disturbances
• General anesthesia
• Infections
• Kidney disease
• Laryngitis
• Liver disorders
• Surgery
• Tumors

As a playful ruse, Plato, in his *Symposium*, afflicted Aristophanes with the hiccoughs—the most famous case in Western literature: "Aristophanes, who was to be the next speaker, comes down with the hiccups. Eryximachus, to his right, suggests he tickle his nostril to sneeze which would cure his hiccups." It apparently did.

Joke: A man is walking up to the doctor's office when a nun comes running out screaming and crying. The man walks in and says, "Doc, what's with the nun?" The doctor says, "Oh, I just told her she's pregnant." The guy says, "The nun's pregnant?" The doctor says, "No. But it certainly cured her hiccups."

The film, *Philadelphia Story*, was shot in eight weeks, and required virtually no retakes. During the scene where James Stewart hiccups when drunk, Cary Grant is looking down and grinning. Since the hiccup wasn't scripted, Grant was on the verge of breaking out laughing and had to compose himself quickly.

Persistent hiccoughs may last for weeks, months, or even years. When hiccoughs are prolonged and severe, therapy may include the administering of certain drugs, inhalation of carbon dioxide, and in stubborn or severe cases are treated with nerve blocks or by surgically cutting the nerve that supplies the diaphragm.

There are rare reports of hiccoughs contributing to death. The most famous is that of Pope Pius XII in 1958, whose death was widely reported to be related to intractable hiccoughs. However, he apparently suffered from recurrent gastritis, which itself could have provoked persistent or intractable hiccups, and he ultimately died of strokes and pneumonia.

Long-term cases have been recorded:

- American Charles Osborne had the hiccoughs for sixty-eight years, from 1922 to 1990, and was entered in the Guinness World Records as the man with the Longest Attack of Hiccups.
- A man who lives in Belfast, Northern Ireland, has had intractable hiccoughs for five years and has had two major operations so far to try to stop them.
- A man in Lincolnshire, England, was reported to have had hiccoughs for at least twenty-two weeks beginning February 2007.
- In January 2007, teenager Jennifer Mee from Florida hiccoughed for five weeks, from January 23, 2007, until February 28, 2007.

Simple hiccoughs will fade away on their own. The many folk remedies for hiccoughs seem to work by blocking the rhythm of the spasms. All of the following have been tried:

Breathing solutions:

- Breathing deeply through the nose, then exhaling slowly through the mouth

- Breathing into a paper bag (in and out, as long as it takes)
- Exhaling air into a small paper bag and immediately re-inhaling that air from it
- Exhaling all the air from one's lungs and holding one's breath while swallowing water or saliva
- Holding one's breath for as long as possible and swallowing at the time one feels the hiccup sensation coming
- Holding one's breath while squeezing one's stomach
- Taking a deep breath through the mouth, leaning forward and pushing down on one's abdomen as long as you can; then slowly exhaling the air through the mouth

Water solutions:
- Bending forward from the waist and drinking water from the wrong side of a glass
- Blocking both ears and drinking six ounces of water without stopping to breathe
- Drinking a glass of water and making sure you gulp only seven times continuously . . . otherwise it won't work
- Drinking a glass of water upside down (This is achieved by holding the glass upright, curling one's lips around the edge of the glass and tilting one's head over.)
- Drinking lots of water and looking to the sky
- Drinking water quickly and burping vigorously
- Drinking a large glass of water without taking a breath
- Gargling with cold water
- Holding one's breath and saying, three times, "Hiccup—sniccup—look up—right up—three drops in a cup—is good for the hiccup"

• Taking a cup of water, and saying: "Hiccups,
Jiccups, Rise up Jacob, Seven gullups in the cup,
Cure Hiccups"

Other methods:
• Blowing up a balloon
• Counting backward from one hundred
• Having someone startle you
• Inducing sneezing
• Plugging your ears with your fingers and drink
something with a straw
• Pulling your tongue out of your mouth as far as you
can and hold it for a couple of seconds
• Smoking a cigarette

In babies, hiccoughs are usually immediately stopped by the suckling reflex, either by breastfeeding or simply by inserting a finger, bottle teat, or dummy into the baby's mouth.

Medications that have been reported to cause hiccoughs include the following:

### Trade/Brand-names

| | | |
|---|---|---|
| Abilify | Digoxin | Medrol |
| Aloxi | Dilantin | Mellaril |
| Ativan | Dopram | Moban |
| Augmentin | Duragesic | Monodox |
| Bactrim | Emend | Morphine |
| Brevital | Exovac | Navane |
| Camptosar | Haldol | Neoral |
| Celontin | Imitrex | Nexium |
| Cerubidine | Invanz | Nicoderm |
| Clopixol | Librium | Orap |
| Clozaril | Lioresal | OxyContin |
| Cytoxan | Lortab | Percocet |
| Decadron | Loxitane | Permax |
| Didronel | Lunesta | Platinol |

## Trade/Brand-names

| | | |
|---|---|---|
| Prezista | Sinemet | Versed |
| Primaxin | Soma | Vicodin |
| Prolixin | Stelazine | Xyrem |
| Reglan | Thorazine | Zarontin |
| Reminyl | Tridione | Zithromax |
| Rocephin | Trilafon | Zofran |
| Romazicon | Tussionex | Zomig |
| Septra | VePesid | |

# Hot Flashes

(Hot Flushes)

Hot flashes (also known as hot flushes) are a symptom of the changing hormone levels that are attributed to menopause. They are typically perceived as a feeling of intense heat with sweating and rapid heartbeat; they may last for a few minutes, and they may be continuous throughout the day. Severe hot flashes can make it almost impossible to get a night's sleep; this can influence mood, concentration, state of mind, and cause other problems. Hot flashes occur when the blood vessels near the skin's surface widen to cool. This leads to the red, flushed look of the face. Some women also develop a rapid heart rate and/or chills. When hot flashes occur at night, they are called "night sweats."

In addition to the hormonal variations of menopause, hot flashes can also be affected by demeanor, habits, and medications (see list on page 241). Eighty-five percent of the women in the United States experience hot flashes as they move toward menopause and for the first year or two after their menstrual periods stop. While most women have mild to moderate hot flashes, about one in ten women experience such intense hot flashes that they request medical assistance.

These flashes usually manifest themselves as sudden, intense, hot feelings on the face and upper body, often attended by a rapid heartbeat and sweating, nausea, dizziness, anxiety, headache, or weakness. Some women experience anxiety or tension just before the hot flash that lets them know what's looming. An episode can last a few seconds, a few minutes, or even an hour. Onsets of these attacks are usually between six and eight in the morning, and between six and ten at night.

When having a hot flash, a woman might experience the following:
- A chilled feeling as the hot flash subsides
- A feeling of mild warmth to intense heat spreading through the upper body and face
- A flushed appearance with red, blotchy skin on the face, neck, and upper chest
- A rapid heartbeat
- Perspiration, mostly on the upper body

They may be accompanied by any or all of the following:
- Accelerated bone loss
- Attention span changes
- Depression and weepiness
- Dryness of eyes and vagina
- Fatigue
- Heart palpitations
- Irritability
- Night sweats
- Reduced libido and interest in sex
- Short-term memory loss
- Sleep disruptions
- Uncharacteristic rage or impatience

Certain triggers may bring hot flashes on more frequently or cause them to be more severe:
- Alcohol
- Caffeine

- Cigarette smoke
- Heat
- Spicy foods
- Stress
- Tight clothing

Medications that can trigger hot flashes include the following:

### Trade/Brand-names

| | | |
|---|---|---|
| Anafranil | Indocin | Orudis |
| Aricept | Intron-A | Pletal |
| Arimidex | Kytril | Ponstel |
| Aromasin | Lamictal | Provera |
| Bumex | Lasix | Sinemet |
| Cardura | Lexapro | Soriatane |
| Casodex | Lotensin | Strattera |
| Celebrex | Lotrel | Synarel |
| Clomid | Lupron | Talwin |
| Demadex | Maxalt | Topamax |
| Dipentum | Meclofenamate | Trelstar |
| Dostinex | Mexitil | Tylenol |
| Eulexin | Mifeprex | Ultram |
| Evista | Migranal | Vitamin $B_{12}$ |
| Exelon | Neoral | Wellbutrin |
| Exovac | Neupro | Zoladex |
| Factive | Noctec | Zyban |
| Feldene | Nolvadex | Zyrtec |
| Femara | Norvasc | |

## Leg Cramps

A muscle cramp is a sudden, uncontrolled, involuntary, sustained tightening (contraction) of one or more of the muscles. It can result in excruciating pain and an inability to use the affected muscles. Night leg cramps, often called a "charley horse," are contractions of the leg muscles, usually in the back of the lower leg (calf). Leg cramps usually last less than a minute, but may last longer before the contraction subsides. They often occur just as one is falling asleep or just when waking up.

The most common cause is exercising: more than usual or differently than usual. Leg cramps are more common in adolescence and in those over age sixty-five.

The precise cause of night leg cramps is not known. Some authorities believe they may be a result of abnormal processing of *electrolyte*s—key elements and chemical substances the body needs for basic functions—by muscles. Almost everyone has occasional leg cramps.

There are some risk factors that are thought to contribute to this condition. They may be a symptom or complication of the following:

- Alcohol use
- Decreased potassium levels
- Dehydration
- Diabetes
- Dialysis treatment
- Excess weight (not necessarily obesity)
- Heavy exercising
- Kidney disease
- Low blood salt
- Medications (see list on pages 243–244)
- Multiple sclerosis
- Muscle overexertion
- Parkinsonism
- Pregnancy
- Prolonged sitting
- Thyroid disorders

Night leg cramps should be distinguished from another common cause of night leg discomfort called *restless legs syndrome*, a condition in which the legs have a creepy, crawly, or fidgety sensation unless you move them (q.v.). This sensation often worsens as night approaches. Restless legs syndrome is a neurologic condition that requires different treatment from that of night leg cramps.

Numerous cures for cramp have been recorded, some with an alleged physical basis, while others are purely magical. Samuel Coleridge Taylor wrote,

> The devil is tying a knot in my leg
> Mark, Luke, and John, unloose it I beg
> Crosses three we make to ease us
> Two for the thieves, and one for Christ Jesus!

A widespread belief in a particular animal bone, carried in the pocket or placed under the pillow, to prevent or cure cramp has a long history, and is still found. In the earliest references, in the sixteenth century, it was a bone from a hare: By the nineteenth century the effective bone was usually the patella, or knuckle-bone of a sheep.

Medications that have been reported to cause leg cramps include the following:

## Trade/Brand-names

| | | |
|---|---|---|
| Agrylin | Evoxin | Oxsoralen |
| Ambien | Exovac | Plavix |
| Atacand | Forteo | Prevacid |
| Atrovent | Foscavir | Proamatine |
| Casodex | Frova | Progesterone |
| Catapres | Glucotrol | Prograf |
| Celebrex | HCTZ | Prostin |
| CellCept | Intron-A | Protonix |
| Claritin | IVIG | Prozac |
| Depakene | Lamictal | Rapamune |
| Depakote | Lipitor | Salagen |
| Desferal | Lyrica | Sular |
| Didronel | Meridia | Synercid |
| Eldepryl | Mirapex | Tenex |
| Estradiol | Natrecor | Teveten |
| Evista | Neoral | Tobrex |

Trade/Brand-names

| | | |
|---|---|---|
| Trelstar | Xopenex | Zonegran |
| Tricor | Xyrem | Zyban |
| Vascase | Zavesca | Zyrtec |
| Vitamin B$_3$ | Zenapax | |
| Wellbutrin | Zomig | |

## Nail Pigmentation

(Melanonychia)

*Nail plate pigmentation* (*melanonychia*) is a common clinical occurrence. The incidence of melanonychia varies according to skin pigmentation, with percentages that may be as high as 77 percent in Blacks over twenty years of age and more in those over fifty years of age but varying with depth of skin color. Ten to 20 percent occur in Asians, and about one percent in Caucasians. These findings present a diagnostic problem because they must be differentiated from subungual melanomas—melanomas beneath the nails—which also occur in older age groups and constitute 50 percent of melanomas in dark-skinned populations.

*Melanonychia striata, or longitudinal melanonychia* (LM), is characterized as either a dark brown or brown-black longitudinal band on a toenail or fingernail. The visual appearance of the fingernails and toenails may suggest an underlying systemic disease. In patients with chronic kidney failure, increased pigment production may cause the distal (end) part of the nail bed to turn brown. In patients with severe kidney disease, the proximal portion of the nail bed (the part closest to the cuticle, also known as the "half-moon") can turn white, obliterating the lunula and giving a half-brown, half-white appearance, also called half-and-half nails.

Most of the medications that can cause pigmented nails are those that are used in the treatment of various malignancies:

## Trade/Brand-names

Adriamycin
Alimta
Alkeran
Blenoxane
Cerubidine
Cytoxan
Decadron
Depakene
Depakote
Depen
Diflucan

Dilantin
Gold
Hycamtin
Hydrea
Idamycin
Methotrexate
Minocin
Neoral
Novantrone
Oxsoralen
Quinora

Rheumatrex
Rimatil
Ruclid
Sumycin
Taxol
Taxotere
Timoptic
Trizivir
Vincasar

## Shivering

(Chills; Hypothermia; Rigors)

> By the time you swear you're his,
> Shivering and sighing,
> And he vows his passion is
> Infinite, undying—
> Lady, make a note of this:
> One of you is lying.
> —Dorothy Parker, "Unfortunate Coincidence"

Shivering is a bodily function in response to early hypo-thermia in warm-blooded animals. (Hypothermia is a condition in which an organism's temperature drops below that required for normal metabolism and bodily functions.) When the body temperature drops, the shivering reflex is triggered. Located in the brain is an area called the primary motor center for shivering. This center becomes switched on when the body temperature falls below a critical temperature level. Muscle groups around the vital organs begin to shake in small movements in an effort to generate warmth by expending energy. Shivering, the involuntary muscular contractions that induce body heat, can also be a response to a fever as a person may feel cold, even though his temperature is already elevated. Chills themselves are temporary, and do not give rise to long-term effects.

The following medical conditions are some of the possible causes of shivering:

- Aging
- Autoimmune disorders
- Cold sensitivity
- Cold sweats
- Cold weather
- Feeling cold
- Fever
- Infections (flu, strep throat, and pneumonia)
- Leukemia and lymphoma
- Menopause
- Panic attacks
- Reactions to medications (see list on page 247)

Other symptoms that might be inaccurately described as "shivering" include the following:

- Seizures
- Spasms
- Tics
- Trembling
- Tremors
- Twitches

The story of King David may be one of the earliest description of a patient affected by shivering. "Now King David was old and stricken in years, and they covered him with clothes, but he gained no warmth." David appears as a rather pathetic old man, shivering uncontrollably in bed, while his court and family maneuver and jockey for position around the dying king.

Superstition says that if a person shivers suddenly and without cause "somebody is walking on that person's grave"—the piece of ground where he or she will someday be buried. It is also believed that sudden shivering means that death is near. Medications responsible for shivering include, among others:

## Trade/Brand-names

| | | |
|---|---|---|
| Amerge | Imitrex | Relpax |
| Anzamet | Lexapro | Romazicon |
| Axert | Luvox | Thiopental |
| Campath | Macrobid | Tylenol |
| Celexa | Maxalt | Ultracet |
| Cymbalta | Miacalcin | Ultram |
| Cytotec | Migranal | Xylocaine |
| Demerol | Paxil | Zenapax |
| Depen | PEG-Intron | Zoloft |
| Diprivan | Precedex | Zomig |
| Effexor | Prostin | Zyprexa |
| Frova | Prozac | |

## Stuttering

(Stammering)

> But he will speak to this nation with stammering lips and in another language.
> —Isaiah, 28:11

Stuttering, also known medically as *dysphemia*, is a speech disorder marked by hesitation and inability to enunciate consonants without spasmodic repetition. This disturbance in the normal fluency of speech does not affect and has no bearing on intelligence. Most stuttering begins in early childhood and studies suggest that about 3 percent of children under the age of five stutter. Males are affected about four times more often than females. Stuttering may be acquired in adulthood as the result of a head injury, tumor, stroke, or drug abuse.

Stuttering—"stammering" in the United Kingdom—occurs in all cultures and races. In 65 percent of cases, there is a family history of the disorder, suggesting a genetic link. Over three million Americans stutter, approximately 1 percent of the population. In certain situations, such as speaking on the telephone, the stuttering might be more severe, depending on the anxiety level related to that activity. Stutterers are more at ease when acting, singing, whispering, or when talking to pets, young children, or themselves.

In addition to personal feelings of shame or anxiety, discrimination is still a significant problem for stutterers. The vast majority of stutterers experience or have experienced bullying, harassment, or ridicule to some degree during their school years, with this trend often carrying over into the workplace. Stuttering is legally classified as a disability in the United States and the United Kingdon.

Stuttering is one of the few disorders that generally get better over time; most children who stutter outgrow it. Even adults who stutter severely in their teens and twenties often overcome stuttering—via speech therapy or on their own—in their thirties or forties.

For centuries stuttering has often featured prominently in both popular culture and in society at large. Some notables who stuttered and went on to have successful lives include the following:

## Actors, Actresses, Singers:
- Nat King Cole
- Rowan Atkinson (Mr. Bean)
- Anthony Quinn
- Bruce Willis
- Carly Simon
- Jimmy Stewart
- Julia Roberts
- Marilyn Monroe

 • Sam Neill
 • Samuel Jackson


## Artists, Composers, Writers, Poets:
 • Lewis Carroll
 • John Updike
 • Miguel de Cervantes
 • Somerset Maugham
 • Virgil, Roman poet
 • Henry James


## Sports Figure:
 • Tiger Woods as a child


## Historical Figures:
 • Isaac Newton
 • King Charles I of England
 • King George VI of England
 • Lenin
 • Napoleon
 • Aesop
 • Aristotle
 • Charles Darwin
 • Claudius
 • Theodore Roosevelt
 • Thomas Jefferson
 • Winston Churchill
 • Balbus Blaesius (Blaesius was a Roman who stuttered so terribly that he became an "exhibit" in a freak show where he was displayed locked in a cage. His last name, Blaesius, is now the Italian word for stuttering.)

Myths surrounding stuttering have created a negative perception of those who stutter and can harm their chances of success in later life:

- Myth: People who stutter are not smart.
  Truth: There is no link between stuttering and intelligence.
- Myth: Stuttering can be "caught" through imitation or by hearing another person stutter.
  Truth: People can't "catch" stuttering
- Myth: Stress causes stuttering.
  Truth: Stress is not the cause; it can, however, aggravate stuttering.
- Myth: Stuttering is caused by emotional or psychological problems.
  Truth: Children and adults who stutter are no more likely to have psychological or emotional problems than children and adults who do not.

In folklore, causes of stuttering have included:

- Allowing an infant to look in the mirror
- Cutting a child's hair before the child spoke his or her first words
- Eating improperly during breastfeeding
- Having too small a tongue
- An imbalance of the four bodily humors: yellow bile, black bile, blood, and phlegm
- The "work of the devil"
- Tickling an infant too much

For centuries, folklore "cures" for stutters have popped up:

- Keeping two or three pea seeds in one's mouth
- Consistently drinking water from a snail shell for the rest of one's life
- Drinking urine of a young mare for thirty days
- Hitting a stutterer in the face when the weather is cloudy

- Speaking with pebbles in the mouth (Demosthenes)
- Strengthening the tongue as a muscle
- Various herbal remedies

Stutterers often have great difficulties saying their own names. Under stress, stutterers tighten the muscles of their vocal cords; thus, stuttering becomes worse when a stutterer is under pressure.

Portrayals of stuttering are seen in the movies *The Right Stuff* (1983), *A Fish Called Wanda* (1988), and *A Family Thing* (1996).

Medications that have been reported to cause stuttering include the following:

### Trade/Brand-names

| | | |
|---|---|---|
| Aminophylline | Neurontin | Sinemet |
| Clozaril | Pertofrane | Xanax |
| Concerta | Prozac | Zoloft |
| Cylert | Risperdal | Zyprexa |
| Lithobid | Ritalin | |

## Yawning

> How weary, stale, flat and unprofitable,
> Seem to me all the uses of this world!
> —William Shakespeare, *Hamlet*, Act 1,
> Scene 2

A yawn is a deep breathing in and breathing out through the mouth and nose associated with weariness, fatigue, exhaustion, inertia, tiredness, lethargy, boredom, and the blahs.

While some popular thoughts believe it to be caused by a lack of oxygen, the specific cause of yawning is not known. Some think that yawning is something that our ancestors used to bare their teeth and intimidate others. Other explanations for this phenomenon are that it is a means of cooling the brain; that it is a lack of oxygen in the blood; that contagious yawning exhibits empathy, or that it is a means of equalizing inner ear pressure. A possible solution to yawning is to breathe through your nose . . .

We do know that yawning is not limited to humans. Cats, dogs, bats, ferrets, even fish yawn, which suggests that yawning is some form of communication. A single shark yawning, especially when it travels in large groups, can set off a yawn reaction in their whole community. A hippo's yawn is not a sign of sleepiness or boredom but is actually a threat gesture. Yawning is the hippo's way of displaying its most fearsome weapons: its long, thick, razor-sharp canine teeth, or tusks, with which it is capable of biting a small boat in half.

Yawning has been associated with ALS (amyotrophic lateral sclerosis), multiple sclerosis, and occasionally with migraine headaches.

## Yawning Trivia:
- Fifty-five percent of people will yawn within five minutes of seeing someone else yawn.
- A phenomenon called "contagious yawning," has been described, in which reading, seeing, hearing, or thinking about someone else yawning causes you to follow suit.
- Blind people yawn more after hearing an audio tape of people yawning.
- Fetuses in the womb yawn.
- In the Hindu world, public yawning was a religious offense.
- Olympic athletes often yawn before competition.
- Pandiculation is the word for stretching and yawning at the same time.
- The average yawn lasts about six seconds.

- Your heart rate can rise as much as 30 percent during a yawn.

## Yawning Superstitions:
- A yawn is a sign that danger is near.
- Counting a person's teeth robs them of one year of life for every tooth counted. This is why some people cover their mouths when they laugh, smile, or yawn.
- If you don't cover your mouth while yawning, the devil will steal your soul. (Estonia)
- A yawn may be a sign that one is afflicted by the evil eye. (Greece)
- If two people are seen to yawn one after the other, the one who yawned last bears no malice toward the one who yawned first.
- In ancient Mayan civilizations, yawning was thought to indicate sexual desires.
- In some countries, it is believed that yawning is caused by someone else talking about you.
- To see others yawning foretells that you will see some of your friends in a miserable state. Sickness will prevent them from their usual labors.
- If you yawn in your dreams, you will search in vain for health and contentment.

Aphorism:

"A yawn is more disconcerting than a contradiction." Mason Cooley

Medications that have been reported to induce yawning include the following:

## Trade/Brand-names

| | | |
|---|---|---|
| Actos | Glucotrol | Requip |
| Amaryl | Glucovance | Robitussin |
| Anafranil | Lexapro | Tambocor |
| Apokyn | Luvox | Tolinase |
| Celexa | Morphine | Tonocard |
| Cymbalta | Orinase | Ultram |
| Diabeta | Paxil | Xylocaine |
| Diamox | Pilocarpine | Zoloft |
| Effexor | Prandin | Zomig |

# GENERAL INDEX

# NAME INDEX